THE CHERRY PIE PARADOX

the CHERRY PIE Paradox

the Surprising PATH to DIET freedom and lasting weight loss

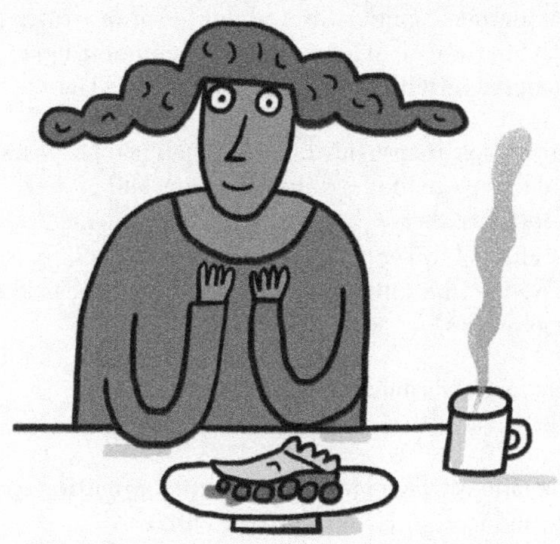

Joy Imboden Overstreet MPH

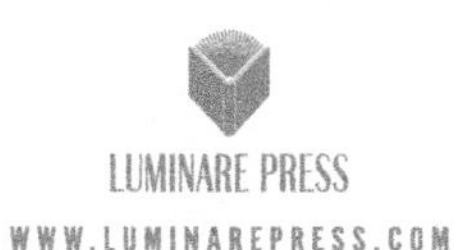

LUMINARE PRESS
WWW.LUMINAREPRESS.COM

The Cherry Pie Paradox:
The Surprising Path to Diet Freedom and Lasting Weight Loss

The resources in this book are provided for informational purposes only and should not be used to replace the specialized training and professional judgment of a healthcare or mental healthcare professional. If you have medical or mental health issues that may be affected by changing your eating practices, please consult a trained professional first. Neither the author nor the publisher can be held responsible for the use of the information provided within this book.

The Cherry Pie Paradox has its foundations in the original Thin Within workshops the author created in Berkeley in 1975. Find more information about her at joyoverstreet.com.

Cover art and illustrations by Kim Murton. More at kimmurton.com.
Production design and interior layout by Claire Flint Last

Printed in the United States of America

Luminare Press
442 Charnelton St.
Eugene, OR 97401
www.luminarepress.com

LCCN: 2021909813
ISBN: 978-1-64388-620-6

To my three children,
Heather Imboden, Ethan Imboden, and Wylie Overstreet,
for decades of unwavering support and laughter.
To Edward, for what you started.
To Werner Erhard, for waking me up.

Table of Contents

PART FOUR: Awaken Your Goal-Mindset

PART FIVE: Traps, Tricks, and Treats

PART SIX: Practice and Persist

Appendices

Begin taking action now, while being neurotic or imperfect, or a procrastinator or unhealthy or lazy or any other label by which you inaccurately describe yourself. Go ahead and be the best imperfect person you can be and get started on those things you want to accomplish before you die.

—Shōma Morita, MD (1874-1938)

READ THIS FIRST

The Cherry Pie Paradox is not a diet. There are no calories, carbohydrates, or points to count, nothing to measure or weigh, no foods to avoid. Besides, who likes to be told they can't have a piece of freshly baked cherry pie? That's why we eventually topple off the regime and the weight returns, along with an extra helping of shame.

The perfect diet that permanently resolves your weight "problem" does not yet exist. If it did, we wouldn't have a multibillion dollar weight-loss industry and more than 70,000 books on the subject. If the perfect diet existed, America's obesity epidemic would disappear; instead more of us are overweight than ever before. Finally, if the perfect diet existed, you would not have picked up this book.

I believe diets are edible Band-Aids, covering the wound without dealing with what's causing it. Diets are for people who want *other* people to tell them what they should and shouldn't eat—so when the diet doesn't work, it's not *their* fault. Diets are for people who believe food is more powerful than they are, so they don the latest diet as if it were a garlic necklace that could ward off vampiric donuts and killer tater tots. Lots of luck with that.

So what *is* this book? It's a door to self-discovery, a road map for action to heal the underlying issues that keep the problem in place, and a step-by-step process to help you reach your natural best size.

The Origins of The Cherry Pie Paradox

Half a lifetime ago, I was a self-styled expert on dieting; I was also an expert at cheating on diets and berating myself for my diet failures.

I had been overweight as a teenager. Even after I lost the extra pounds, the emotional scars from that episode and from our fat-shaming culture lingered. I became hypervigilant about my weight and spent the next twenty years tinkering with the latest diets to prevent a relapse.

Then, my husband died of cancer in mid-1974, leaving me with our two little ones to raise alone, as well as many *feelings*. Some of those feelings were not surprising—grief over the loss, and anxiety as I contemplated a scary future as a single mom with few readily marketable skills. What I didn't expect was a tsunami of *unacceptable* feelings: anger that Edward had ruined my perfect life plan; guilt that I hadn't been more loving and caring in the final year of his life; and crippling shame about being obsessed with something so shallow as what I weighed, when my kids had lost the father who adored them.

Eating helped me manage those feelings—or so I told myself. But the more I ate, the more I obsessed about my weight. Every night, I designed a new diet for myself, and within 24 hours I had cheated on it. I hated myself for being so out of control.

I hit bottom six months after Edward's death. I sat on the couch, wallowing in self-pity, and mortified by my petty concerns. In my left hand, I held a jar of crunchy peanut butter and in my right, a large spoon. Yet another diet book lay open on my lap. The floor was littered with tear-soaked tissues and travel brochures from a friend who thought it would help if I got away.

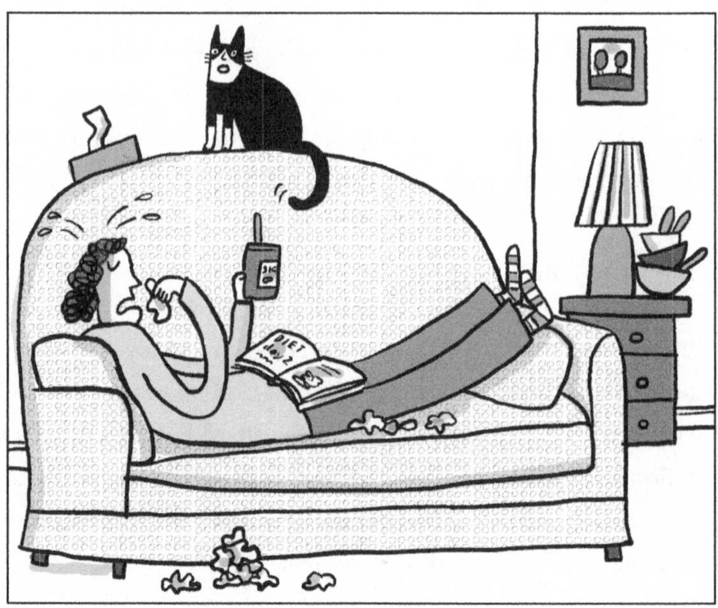

But a trip would be pointless, because wherever I went, there I would be. And I'd be eating.

Suicide seemed like the only other way to get away from myself. I couldn't figure out how to kill myself in a tidy way, so I went straight to imagining myself dead, stretched out lifeless on the couch. (I've always had an active imagination.) Even though I adored Heather, then 6, and Ethan, 3, more than anything in the world, my thinking was so warped I failed to recognize my death would make them orphans.

Continuing to spin my tragic fantasy… the coroner would arrive to examine the body. He would lift my bulky sweater and… oh my God, he would see my hidden fat. That did it. Suicide was out. The mortifying truth: vanity saved my life.

> [Today, I can laugh at my melodrama. At the time, however, I felt the kind of claustrophobic desperation of a passenger who's strapped into their seat in a flaming airplane hurtling towards earth. I remember too well the anguish and crushing shame. So if you are in that place, I hope you can get professional help.]

I threw the diet book on the floor with the rest of the litter. If I was going to live, I had to leap off the diet hamster wheel. Heather and Ethan might end up with a fatter mom, but I had to find some other way to regain my sanity—let the tortilla chips fall where they may.

A concerned friend, Chérie Carter-Scott, stepped in to help me lift my gaze beyond the agonies of the moment. She used her coaching skills to ask questions about my vision for the next part of my life. But all I could think about was losing weight.

"What if the obstacle—your weight problem—is the path?" she asked. "Instead of shoving down those feelings with food, denying that you're eating what you're eating, and beating yourself up for all your diet failures, how about letting what you call your "problem" be your teacher?

Could you learn something by being present to your experience in the moment, as painful as it might seem?"

I had to admit that everything I'd tried had only made me more miserable. What did I have to lose?

I would start by trying to pay more attention to what I was eating and how I was talking to myself. I decided to enlist all five of my senses in becoming more mindful of the food that somehow (*mystery of mysteries!*) arrived in my mouth.

The paradoxical effect of such focus was that I began to feel more hopeful and more in control of myself.

And then a few days later something happened that shifted *everything*.

Breakfast with an Alien

I had delivered my kids to the home of another parent from our children's nursery school for a morning play date. Carol was just sitting down to breakfast and invited me to join her.

I expected some coffee and maybe a piece of toast. Wrong. Carol's breakfast was cherry pie, fresh from her oven. My brain spun. Pie for breakfast?

"Oh, no thanks," I said primly, "I don't eat pie; I'm trying to lose weight." I grabbed a cup off the counter. "I'll take some coffee though. Black."

"You sure? It's a pretty fine pie, if I say so myself." She cut herself a large piece and transferred it to her plate, red juices flowing. My salivary glands sprang into action.

In my world of nutritional Dos and Don'ts, pie was a definite Don't. But what really got my attention was who was eating this rich breakfast: tiny, slender Carol.

We sat ourselves in the breakfast nook, Carol with her pie and me with my coffee, trying not stare as she savored each bite. Then, with half of the wedge still on her plate, she patted her tummy with a gesture of satisfaction, pulled the garbage can over to the table and tossed the rest of the piece.

Whaaaat? Perfectly good food! Cherry pie! Just tossed! In the garbage!

It took all my restraint not to dive into the can after the half-eaten slice. If I were a cartoon figure, smoke would have poured out my ears. Carol's behavior called into question everything I'd believed about dieting and being slim.

I tried to make sense of what I had witnessed. I had a vague memory of reading an article that described two categories of thin people—"true thins" and "fat thins." *True thins* were slim on the outside and never worried about their weight or what they ate. This was Carol. *Fat thins* might or *might not* be carrying extra weight, but nevertheless obsessed about what they ate and were unable to shake their "fat" self-image. Even though I might look slim enough to others, I was undeniably a *fat thin*.

The humanist psychologist Abraham Maslow revolutionized therapeutic practice in the early 1960s with his novel approach to mental health. He believed that studying the behavior of healthy, productive, mature individuals provided more useful information about psychological health than the prevailing practice of studying those with emotional issues.

Had I been relying on advice from diet experts who had only studied people with weight problems? At best, these folks had lost weight and become slimmer on the *outside*, but my hunch was that many remained *fat* in their heads, doomed like me to chronic weight worries. What if I looked instead for guidance from natural slimness masters—*true thins* like Carol?

This was my eureka moment. I knew that nothing in life is fixed, and that within each so-called absolute is the seed of its opposite. The Taoist yin-yang symbol is a perfect expression of that truth. You can't know hot without knowing cold, light without dark. I just had to discover, awaken, and nurture the *thin* seed that had to be lurking somewhere inside my *fat* head. [I use the words "thin" and "fat" as shortcut terms, but I attach no particular number of pounds or body mass index to either word. Insert your own personal definitions or phrases. See chapter 1, The F-Word, for a deeper discussion of these loaded terms.]

I decided to study how *true thins* related to food and their bodies, comparing these discoveries with my own thinking and behavior.

The next few weeks were intense. I watched other people of all shapes and sizes as they ate, and I quizzed them about their attitudes toward food. I also became my own lab rat, observing my behavior as objectively as I could. I took voluminous notes on what I ate, how my body sensed hunger and fullness, what situations made me want to eat, and how many self-serving excuses I created for eating when I wasn't hungry.

Most importantly, I searched for evidence of my own inner thin self. Whenever I caught a glimpse of what I began to call my thin behavior, I heaped myself with praise. Sometimes I pretended I was Carol (WWCD-What Would Carol Do?) to give that inner *thin* self a workout.

To my amazement, the extra pounds began to come off. My depression lifted, and I felt a new surge of energy.

One night I awoke with the name "Thin Within" lighting up my brain. It perfectly matched what I wanted to *be*. And sharing this method of inner exploration with other fed-up dieters was what I wanted to *do*. [Quick aside here. As much as I loved this name in 1975, today the word "thin" is no longer alluring to most of us.]

I had no idea if the enormous shift I'd experienced in my own relationship to food and my weight would work for anyone else, so I drafted a series of classes. Five women in the neighborhood volunteered to be my guinea pigs for the first Thin Within seminars. We launched in my living room in May of 1975.

To my astonishment, over the next few weeks all of us lost weight and everyone loved the process of discovery. We marveled at our creative excuses and the myriad ways we'd found to avoid taking responsibility for our behavior. It became clear that weight problems don't erupt out of nowhere; they're often a solution to other issues with long-buried histories—birth-family dynamics, trauma, and cultural pressures.

Over the next few months, I taught additional groups, refining and adding to the course material. By October I knew the Thin Within program would soon outstrip my ability to manage it by myself, especially as a single parent. (As my sanity returned, so did my desire to be the attentive parent my kids deserved, thank goodness.)

In late fall, I took on a partner, Judy Wardell Halliday, who had experienced similar weight struggles. She had a background as a psychiatric nurse and we seemed to have complementary strengths. I acknowledge with gratitude that without Judy's enormous contributions, Thin Within would have died of my exhaustion. Instead, it thrived in the San Francisco Bay Area over the next few years, enabling hundreds of participants to make peace with food and their bodies.

In 1980, I sold my share of Thin Within to Judy and returned to school for a graduate degree in public health. Shortly after, Judy became a born-again Christian and began altering the program to be Bible-based.

Since then, many weight-loss programs have adopted and adapted a number of Thin Within's revolutionary principles. *The Cherry Pie Paradox* maintains the framework of my original step-by-step transformation process, significantly updated with lots of new material I've incorporated from four decades of experience in Asian mindfulness traditions, new developments in neuroscience and the psychology of behavior change.

Today, given the strides made in body positivity (appreciating our bodies no matter their size or shape), some writers would retire the words "fat" and "thin" because they refer to appearance, not substance. However, political correctness aside, these terms refuse to die in our trash-talking minds when we look in the mirror or try on a new outfit, so I use them where necessary. Please understand, I am talking about your thinking and behavior, not your appearance.

And, in case you're wondering, I have not dieted since 1975 and remain slim. If you offered me a piece of cherry pie for breakfast (and if I were hungry), I would accept with pleasure.

Is This Book Right for You?

Of course, I think *everyone* would benefit from a healthier, more satisfying relationship with food and their bodies by following these practices. However, what will be most helpful to you depends on whether your concerns are relatively recent or have been ongoing for decades, and whether you want to lose weight or just make peace with food and the body you have.

- **If you've been a chronic yo-yo dieter,** you will have accumulated a lot of negative mental baggage. Your weight issues have become a problem of ***over-attention***—listening too much to the trash-talker in your head, and of ***under-attention***—not being mindful of your body or your food. You'll need time, focus, and patience to free yourself for good. It's important to do all the exercises sequentially.
- **If you never worried about your weight... until one day in middle age** you could no longer zip your jeans, or the doctor announced your health would improve if you lost weight, or you looked down at your expanded waist and wondered, *What the hell happened here?* You had always thought of yourself as a "thin" person. This is a problem of ***under-attention***—ignoring what your mouth and body have been trying to tell you. The eating, hunger, and body awareness exercises ("SuperTools") should reawaken your inner sylph.
- **If you simply want to feel good about your body as it is, whatever your weight, this process can help you too.** It's tragic to dislike the only body you'll ever receive. You have a problem of ***over-attention*** to the trash-talker in your head. I hope some of the mindfulness exercises and SuperTools help you befriend the body you have and allow you to enjoy the foods you choose to eat without guilt or shame.

If you have a medical condition that requires you to avoid certain foods, eat frequent meals, or follow a special schedule, or if you have issues with bulimia or anorexia, please follow your doctor's orders first.

This book provides an experiential exploration that requires your open-minded curiosity and willingness to experiment. You can follow the program whether you're carnivorous, gluten-free, vegetarian, vegan,

Vietnamese, Mexican, or Bulgarian—because it's about how you eat, why you eat, and how much you eat, not *what* you eat.

You will experience shifts in many dimensions:

- **In perspective:** from harsh judge to curious researcher, from fighting a "weight problem" to implementing a freedom project
- **In self-image:** from "fat" to "right-size-for-me"
- **In self-talk:** from making excuses to getting results
- **In habits:** from self-defeating behaviors to empowering choices
- **In awareness:** from mindless stuffing to developing a discriminating palate
- **In attitudes toward food:** from tempting hazard to sensory pleasure
- **In relationship to your body:** from out of touch to attentive appreciation

Your future is created in the present moment. Yesterday's half-gallon of ice cream is in the past and tomorrow's buffet extravaganza has not yet happened. What gets in the way of being here and now is your constantly yammering internal critic and other ancient junk—unexamined habits, tired excuses, squashed emotions and dreams, and your self-limiting stories about who you think you are.

The present moment is your only opportunity to choose more wisely, and you have it within your power do so. You deserve to eat what you love and love what you eat. You deserve freedom from disquieting or oppressive thoughts and an end to hostilities between you and your body. You deserve to live in a body you treasure, even if occasionally it might need a fresh coat of paint. You deserve to leave this problem in the dust, so you can fulfill your real purpose in life.

You can do this.

How To Use This Book

The Cherry Pie Paradox is a sequential process of self-discovery. It's an action-oriented approach to healing your relationship to food and your body—a rewarding practice that becomes a permanent way of life.

You'll find fresh perspectives to consider, daily practices to cement your healthier habits, and prompts to guide you through written reflections, eating experiments, guided meditations, and other activities. I offer five SuperTools that are core elements of this practice, and many others that you'll want to adapt to your personal preferences and circumstances. Many can be applied to improve other sticky situations that life tosses your way.

The book is in six parts. The chapters build on each other, so work through them in order. Some will be worth re-reading as your awareness expands with practice.

Part One: The Groundwork. What you need to know before digging into the process.

Part Two: Start Where You Are. What's true right now? You begin to collect some data on your current eating habits.

Part Three: The Enemy in Your Head. Negative thought patterns are keeping you stuck in a vicious cycle. Sunlight is the best disinfectant.

Part Four: Awaken Your Goal-Mindset. What does it mean to be someone who is free of weight worries? Find and strengthen that person within yourself.

Part Five: Traps, Tricks, and Treats. How to handle everyday perils and pleasures.

Part Six: Practice and Persist. Tips for maintaining your practice for life.

Appendix: In case you don't have internet access this is where you'll find copies of questionnaires, charts, and transcripts for the guided meditations, as well as credits and additional resources. However, all this material is on my website in a private folder just for you (joyoverstreet.com/pie), organized by chapter. The meditation transcripts are included as a last resort because they're far more effective when you're guided through them. Besides, most people cannot read when their eyes are shut.

What You Will Need

- **The boundless curiosity and dispassionate attitude of a scientist.** Instead of backing away from what you fear could be a bottomless pit, step forward with a mind open to making fresh discoveries about yourself. After all, who is a more fascinating creature than *you?*

  Like a scientist who has ideas, theories, and hypotheses, you'll be trying a variety of experiments. Like a scientist, you'll observe the results of your experiments, doing your best to suspend judgment. Like a scientist, when an experiment doesn't pan out, you don't toss your microscope out the window. Instead, you get curious and explore further. *Hmm,* you ask yourself, *what happened here and why?* You make adjustments and carry on. Failure is a waystation full of valuable information, not the end point.

- **Loving kindness toward yourself.** This is deep work. You will discover some things about yourself that may displease you. Congratulations! You are human. The inner critic is our worst enemy. Instead of letting her run amuck every time you observe your faults and failures, imagine you're the parent of a darling toddler whom you love unconditionally, despite her occasional temper tantrums or drawing on the wall with permanent markers. Your love never wavers because you know she's doing her best for her level of development. You too are doing your best, and you're learning.

- **Notebook and pen.** (✏📖) I prefer the flexibility of blank pages to a formatted workbook, so get yourself a medium-sized spiral-bound notebook. Spiral binding allows you to fold it back on itself so it takes less space on the table. The A5 sized (approximately 6" x 8") notebooks are small enough to fit in your bag, but capacious enough to hold many words. I love the smooth paper and dot-grid layout in those made by two different Japanese companies, Miliko and Mnemosyne. Both available online.

Your notebook will sit open beside you every time you eat, allowing you to take notes in the moment. What you write will be a mix of food diaries, prompt responses, brain dumps, and jotting down beliefs, excuses and ahas as they happen. Don't worry about eloquence—lists and sentence fragments will do. Journaling is an opportunity to excavate those subconscious saboteurs ruling your behavior so you can deal with them, *mano a mano*. You'll be surprised by the insights that emerge alongside the blah blah blah. You may even find intriguing messages in your dreams.

You should review your notebook entries every few days, looking for patterns and new insights, especially when things seem to go wrong. Mistakes are the best teachers, so rejoice and make note of how you might adjust the experience or act to prevent a recurrence.

➤ **Internet access.** Bookmark joyoverstreet.com/pie in your web browser now. It's a private folder just for readers of this book. The materials mentioned below are there, organized by chapter.

- **Guided meditations [💬 👂].** When you see the talk bubble + ear symbols, that means you should put down the book and allow yourself to be led through the meditation. (There are nine of them sprinkled through the book.) For the most powerful effect, I recommend you LISTEN and let yourself be guided, rather than read the transcripts. Your troublesome *thinking* mind is thus bypassed, allowing memories and images to pop up before you can judge or squash them as irrelevant. In order to make new discoveries your imagination needs the freedom to roam.

- **Questionnaires and blank forms for charting your progress.** You can download whatever copies you need.

- **Positivity partners you can share the process with.** It really *really* helps to "work the program" with others. They can hold you accountable for doing the assignments, be there to share discoveries and stuck places. You can help each other let go of shame, and you can laugh together as you recognize you're not alone in your folly. Other people's stories open our minds to our own personal blind spots. (Sharing was a super-important part of the original Thin Within workshop series.)

  If you want to organize your own support and accountability group for working through the book, I recommend a group of at least four people for a wider variety of experiences. For ideas on conducting your group, check out my website, where you can also subscribe to my weekly newsletter.

- **The willingness to practice. *And the patience to persist.*** Every baby step forward will reap benefits down the road. Remember, you spent years shaping your negative self-image and counterproductive habits. New neuroscience discoveries tell us that our brains remain malleable throughout life; your self-identity can and will shift depending on the behaviors you repeat. So as you choose more mindful and constructive behaviors day by day, you will begin to see yourself as a person who is no longer run by food and your weight. This is how you become a healthy eater for life.

Your daily practice will ask you to:

- Stay curious; maintain a "beginner's mind"
- Tell the truth about what you're eating
- Be present to your body, so you can act on its hunger and fullness signals
- Be present to your food, so you can savor what's delicious and leave what isn't
- Recognize when your stories, beliefs, and counterproductive habits are running the show

- Take responsibility for your power to make choices
- Acknowledge and affirm every instance of supportive behavior
- Treat all "failures" as learning experiences
- Use your positivity partners to stay on track with frequent check-ins
- Treat yourself and your body with the same respect, patience, and compassion you would your dearest friend

So, let's get started!

✏📖 **Prompt: Fill out the "Before" questionnaire.** It's in Appendix A and also available online as a downloadable Word document on my website joyoverstreet.com/pie, giving you space for your answers to expand as you write. Once you complete it, set it aside and don't look at it again until you've done the "After" questionnaire some weeks or months from now. You can then compare what has shifted.

PART ONE

The Foundation

What you need to know before starting this practice. Coming to terms with the "F-word." Where does your responsibility begin and end? Calibrating your essential tools. Adjusting your attitude and expectations.

1

Coming to Terms with the "F-word"

Sticks and stones may break my bones, but words have also hurt me.
—Ellen B., Thin Within participant

Let's talk about the F-word. Not the four-letter F-word. The three-letter F-word. *Fat.*

In 1975, when I created the original Thin Within workshops, American culture held the words "fat" and "thin" very differently than we do today.

To be "fat" in the mid-twentieth century was a terrible thing, especially for women. My friends and I lived by the daily report from our bathroom scales. If the readout was up by even two pounds, it was *A-ooga! A-ooga! All hands on deck!* Get out the latest diet, the little cans of Slim Fast glurp, the exercise bands, the Ayds weight-loss candies. (Yes, candies for weight loss—they didn't work, but were damn tasty).

I remember how I despaired when I read *The Thin Book by a Formerly Fat Psychiatrist* by Dr. Theodore Isaac Rubin (1966). His opening chapter, I kid you not, is titled "Fatness is a Sickness." He says,

> *Being fat is a sickness. For our purposes, you're fat and sick if you're at all overweight. This applies whether you're mildly sick, i.e., 3 or 4 pounds overweight, or deathly sick, i.e., some 75 or more pounds overweight. Like many sicknesses, neglect will result in the acute becoming chronic and the benign becoming malignant... Fat people are anxiety ridden and handle their anxiety through overeating.*

Today, we recognize how hurtful the label "fat" can be. And as for "thin," what does that even mean? Slim? Slender? Carrying 20 (40, 60, 80, 100) pounds less than you do today? To someone struggling with anorexia, scrawny might feel too fat.

Even in the late 1970s when "thin" was what everyone wanted to be, we left the definitions of fat and thin to our Thin Within participants. Most wanted to lose weight, but in every class we had several who were at an acceptable weight, yet they still felt fat inside—they could never let down their guard against the magnetic power of food, could never enjoy a dessert without guilt, and still could not accept, much less appreciate, the bodies they had.

In updating Thin Within's powerful practices for *The Cherry Pie Paradox*, I wanted to replace the words *fat* and *thin* with terms that felt less judgmental, because no one deserves to be judged on size. So in this book, the term "fat" represents not just unwanted adipose tissue, it's also a filter through which many with weight problems see the world. I use the term "fat-mindset" to encompass a set of counterproductive beliefs, stories and excuses; a certain amount of denial; and a disconnection from both the body and the sensory experience of eating.

In contrast, some of us imagine that "thin" or "slim" is some kind of nirvana, where you become a Boston marathoner, irresistible to potential sex partners, successful in business, and you live happily ever after surrounded by puppies, kittens and rainbows. Sure.

Like many of you, I no longer find the word *thin* alluring. What I once called "thin-mindset" I'm now calling "goal-mindset."

Goal-mindset is the positive self-image that motivates you to keep going. You define it for yourself—your intended weight, level of health and fitness, relationship to food and your body, etc. Goal-mindset brings forth the skillful attitudes, beliefs, and behaviors that will make your goal a physical reality.

Ultimately this is a healing process and life practice. Yes, we'll cheer when you reach your weight goal, but keep your eyes on the real prize: an ongoing peaceful and appreciative relationship with food and your body, so you can leave your weight worries behind and get on with the important work of your life.

REMEMBER THIS

- Fat and thin are just words. You know who you want to be.
- The real prize is the freedom to get on with the important work of your life.

2

An Attitude Adjustment

From "Problem" to "Project"

This process should not be a dreary slog. It requires attention, yes, but it's also full of delightful surprises and pleasures. I hope you find it en*lighten*ing in all senses of the word—not just in how you deal with your relationship to food and your body, but also how you approach other challenging areas of your life.

If you've been talking about your weight "problem" for years, your enlightening attitude adjustment starts here, with the word *problem*. *Problem* brings to mind a situation that is heavy, stuck, unwanted. Just like those extra pounds. A millstone. As you can imagine, we're daunted by the inertia of a millstone, so instead we make half-assed efforts, or we give up before we even begin.

Instead, let's use the word *problem* only for identification purposes—what is the situation that needs fixing? Once it's identified, you can plan your next steps. At this point, the problem becomes a *project*, like remodeling your bathroom. Now, as a project, it's actionable, one step at a time.

Defining the project not only helps you define your action steps, it also keeps you on track by excluding distractions. If I want to remodel my bathroom, shopping for a new mattress is off purpose.

Name Your Project and Your Why

So, let's reframe your weight problem. From now on, it's a *project*. You can call it whatever speaks to you—your "get slim 'n' trim project," your "reclaim my energy and sanity project," or your "I love me as I am" project. *You* decide what outcome you intend. It is not a number on the scale; it's a positive vision that compels you forward. I used to call it my *freedom project*—freedom from extra pounds and freedom from obsessing about food and my body flaws (flaws as perceived by me, anyway).

You may have an idea of your "right size" that you're shooting for, but more importantly, do you have a vision of your *why*? *Why* do you want to change? Put another way, losing X pounds or becoming less obsessed is not actually an end point; it's an obstacle you've removed ***so that*** you have the freedom to do something more meaningful. Your *so that*___ is your real *why*.

Even my bathroom remodel project had a *why*. I knew that a new sink stand and light fixture wouldn't change my life. But I had a vision of the end in mind— a bathroom that worked better, *so that* I could more easily get ready for events of the day ahead.

Do not skip this exercise.

Prompt: My _____ Project. Name your project and your *why*. Close your eyes and dare to imagine yourself having completed this project. The more compelling your vision, the more you'll be inspired to keep going when you feel discouraged. What will that look like? How will you feel? What do you hope to gain as a result of completing your project? (Examples: The ability to enjoy a long hike or play tag with your kids? The confidence to apply for a better job?) Take out your notebook and write about this.

Now fill in the blanks: "I'm completing my _____ Project *so that* I can_____, and_____, and _____."

And finally: Ask yourself, *Is anything stopping me from starting in on my why today (regardless of my size)?*

How Will You Measure Success?

If you're expecting the angels to sing when you complete your ___ Project, I'm here to tell you you're going to be disappointed. Even if the angels do sing, it will be a short song, and then you'll be on to the next thing. If you're trying to free yourself from a lot of weight or years of obsessive thinking, it could be a looong wait for those angels to show up. Instead, please consider the importance of celebrating along the way as you reach certain personal milestones. Look deep and consider what modest successes you hope to achieve during the process. Here are some ideas:

- I can say no to second helpings, despite wanting to please my hosts.
- I kept my weight stable over the holidays.
- I ate a piece of pie without feeling any guilt.
- I throw away the last bite of food on my plate as a habit.
- My jeans feel looser.
- When I'm complimented on how good I'm looking, I actually agree.
- I now pause before eating to breathe and feel grateful, instead of diving in.
- I no longer eat standing up in the kitchen.

Prompt: Write a list of the modest successes that will indicate you're making progress along the journey. To start, think about the small ways you've felt flummoxed in previous wars with your weight, and what changes would let you know you're on the right path this time.

Spectator or Participant?

Your Project is a hero's journey. You (our hero) realize dieting and obsessing are not working for you, so you're called to action.

But, there be dragons! You feel the hot breath of your fears, past failures, old wounds, the unknown. Fortunately, your fairy godmother is giving you a map and some new dragon-fighting tools, should you dare to implement them. You screw up your courage, step forward, and look the dragons in the eye. They are not used to such scrutiny, and they begin to shrink. Battles and skirmishes occur, some of which you lose (temporarily), but gradually you get stronger and the dragons get weaker. Some skitter back into their caves, never again to emerge; others become downright funny, and you find it hard to believe they once seemed so scary. Eventually you emerge victorious!

Remember, heroes are not spectators. They participate fully. To get the results you want, you cannot watch from the sidelines, you must get down on the playing field.

I know exactly what your devious little mind is saying right now: "I'll read this book and *think about* whether or not it makes sense to me—maybe do a couple of the exercises *to see if I like them*." Then, when you don't see instant results, you put the book aside. "This will never work for me," you tell yourself. And you get to be right. Again. But you're also cheating yourself.

Every step of this process requires *action* on your part. The lessons are meant to be experienced first-hand, and the discoveries made by you in your own life. *Reading* about and *hearing* about won't cut it. My son used to give me blow-by-blow accounts of his favorite movies, and couldn't understand why I didn't feel the magic. Or consider the difference between reading a recipe for crème brulée versus cracking the top with your spoon and slipping the creamy custard into your mouth. It's like that. You can't just watch and wait for proof without doing the work. If you put these tools into regular practice and patiently persevere, baby step by baby step, you will reach your goal.

Practice, Practice, Practice! It's how you get to Carnegie Hall, and it's also how you get to live as a fit, slim, free, healthy (insert your word) person for the rest of your life.

Most athletes and musicians practice every day. So do yogis and others who follow a spiritual practice of meditation and prayer. Like yoga, mindful eating is a life practice. It's what we do regularly over an extended period of time, which deepens the connection to our experience and expression of aliveness.

The journey begins. I hope you chose to be a participant.

• • • • • REMEMBER THIS • • • • •

- A *problem* weighs you down; a *project* is actionable, step by step.
- Action is key. Be a participant, not a spectator.

3

Is Your Body Shape Your Fault?

In life our first job is this—to divide and distinguish things into two categories: externals I cannot control, but the choices I make with regard to them I do control.

—Epictetus

It's a waste of emotional energy to fault and shame ourselves for factors we have no control over. Let's lighten your emotional burden and point the blame elsewhere for once. Here are some factors that are not of your own making.

You Are Your Parents' Child

Genetics. The shape of your nose or your hands, the relative size of your boobs or your butt, your talent for music or math—these were determined by your DNA when sperm and egg met. There's no use berating yourself for any of this, any more than it's useful to berate gravity when the apple falls off the tree and bonks you on the head.

Your family of origin. You were raised by people who created an environment you accepted as the norm because it was all you knew. Like water is to a fish, it was invisible to you. However, those early years shaped your version of reality—what kind of people raised you, where they lived, how much money they had, their level of education, what they believed, what they expected of you, their food preferences, eating habits, cultural traditions, on and on. You were more or less oblivious to the uniqueness of your reality until you got out into the world and realized, "Oh! Not everyone eats donuts and a Coke for breakfast." "Who knew Brussels sprouts could be tasty!" "You mean I don't have to eat everything on my plate?"

This last one was a huge aha! for me. My chunky mother was a big proponent of the Clean Plate Club, for herself and for us kids. As she finished off anything we left uneaten, she would sometimes brag, "I'll eat anything that isn't spoiled; I'm a human garbage pail." Wanting to be a good parent myself, I became the Human Garbage Pail of Spruce Street—a startling realization that surfaced one day when I was doing a brain dump in my journal.

In later chapters, you'll get to bring fresh eyes to these early influences and determine which ones are supportive of your goals, and which ones are holding you back.

You Live in America

Bombardment by junk food. Producers of processed foods make the highest profit margins. Walk into most supermarkets and notice what is most prominently featured—you'll see a sea of candy, chips, cookies, soft drinks at every check stand and end-aisle display. Unless you shop in a natural food store, a far greater percentage of square footage is taken up with processed foods than raw ingredients (and quite honestly there's a lot of junk at Whole Foods too—just more expensive). Then, turn on the TV in the evening, when you're most vulnerable to snacking. You're bombarded with commercials for snack food, fast food outlets, and drugs (many necessitated by our terrible food habits). As Bee Wilson writes in *The Way We Eat Now,* "Since the birth of farming ten thousand years ago, most humans haven't been hunters, but never before have we been so consistently pursued by our own food supply. The calories hunt us down even when we are not looking for them."

When was the last time you saw a TV commercial for carrots, broccoli or apples? I rest my case.

A culture of body shaming. Americans are obsessed with the human body and its natural functions. Despite the prevalence of pornography and cooking shows, deep down many of us still hold puritanical views about lust and gluttony. Think about it: in the Bible, the very first sin was eating! How many times have you heard that a particular food is "sinfully rich" or "devilishly delicious?" as if only a sinful person would eat it. *Godly* people exercise restraint over these base desires, so if you're plump, you're wearing your moral failings all over your body. During both World Wars, because of international food shortages, being thin was considered a patriotic duty; Americans were encouraged to support the troops overseas by eating less. "Lay your double chin on the altar of liberty," said one New Jersey newspaper.

The diet industry. Between the diet books, the special programs, the special foods, and the phone apps, we're pumping billions of dollars into the diet industry every year. If you read up on the history of America's love affair with dieting, you realize that it's been going on since the middle of the 19th century, when Sylvester Graham and William Kellogg opened a sanitarium in Battle Creek, Michigan, promoting an ascetic way of eating as a cure for all ills, physical and moral. Many of the diet fads we have today are sons, cousins, and sometimes twins of diet fads that have been circulating in our culture for more than a hundred years.

Even if you have zero interest in losing weight, there are countless other ways to restrict your eating (aka *to diet*) and obsess about your food. Off the top of my head: steer clear of gluten, meat, dairy, sugar, salt, the nightshade family, carbohydrates or "white" foods, additives of any kind, foods low in fiber or nutrients, foods that aren't organic or locally sourced, foods not blessed by your religious faith. Also, do not eat after 6 in the evening or before 10 in the morning. Drink 8 glasses of water a day, but not as diet soda. Don't mix protein and carbs in the same meal…What have I missed?

No wonder you're a little crazy! As Virginia Sole-Smith says in her fascinating book, *The Eating Instinct: Food Culture, Body Image, and Guilt in America,* "For too many of us, food feels dangerous. We parse every bite we eat as good or bad and judge our own worth accordingly."

All this is to say—America's obesity epidemic is not your personal fault. We're drowning in a toxic sea of temptations, food fads, unrealistic expectations, and shame for falling short. Strengthen yourself against this onslaught by becoming aware of the cultural forces you're up against. Get curious about the influences in your own environment and think of steps you can take to inoculate yourself going forward.

The following two prompts aren't essential assignments, but should you decide to do them, you'll find them eye-opening.

✏📖 **Prompt: TV commercial log.** If you're a regular television viewer, for a couple of evenings keep a tally of the commercials. How many for food, drink, or diets? Specifically, what ones? When one runs, do you suddenly feel an urge to eat something? If you don't snack, do you feel like you're missing out?

✏📖 **Prompt: Grocery store survey.** Explore the store where you usually shop for groceries. What kinds of foods are most prominent, displayed on the ends of aisles or by the check stands? How many aisles are given over to candy, snacks and highly processed foods, nutritional supplements, soft and other sweetened drinks? How many to basic ingredients like meat, fish, vegetables, fruit, beans, grains, bread, dairy?

• • • • • REMEMBER THIS • • • • •

- You are not to blame for your DNA, the family who raised you, the greedy food industry, or American culture.
- Many life circumstances are beyond our control.
- Become aware of them. Your power lies in how you respond.

4

What *Is* Your Responsibility?

You were not tied to the bedpost and force-fed that jumbo bag of potato chips. (And who put them in your shopping cart?) Your mother isn't watching to see if you finished every crumb on your plate. Your host won't like you more just because you took seconds on her casserole. In other words, *you* ate that thing.

The "devil" that made you do it sits between your ears—it's your mind. It's your mind that wanders off while you're eating, so you won't notice what or how much you're putting in your mouth. Your mind doesn't pay attention to your body's hunger or fullness signals and creates plausible reasons why you deserve to eat that big hunk of chocolate cake. Your mind suggests eating those Cheetos will make you less anxious, squash your anger, or help you avoid a difficult conversation. Your mind whispers that you're doomed to be fat, so eating one more won't make a difference.

Once you become aware of your mind's role in the matter, you can begin to rein it in and make wiser choices. As James Baldwin once said, "Not everything that is faced can be changed, but nothing can be changed until it is faced."

The Dream of Quick and Easy

Many people who want to lose weight are discouraged if the pounds don't melt quickly and easily. Maybe you've been on diets where the first 20 pounds dropped off in a month. It could happen, but for most folks, it's a slow and steady process. This is preferable, because if you lose weight too fast, your body freaks out and thinks it's starving, so when you quit the diet, it grabs on to those calories and slaps them back on your thighs with a vengeance. So, patience, my friend, patience. A half-pound a week is 26 pounds a year—pounds that will stay gone.

As for easy—who wouldn't prefer a magic cure? That's why we see so many clickbait ads on the internet to "burn unwanted fat." My magic cure involved a body-sized fat-cutter. I'd lie down on a countertop like a big blob of dough, and with the press of a button, a cookie cutter the exact shape of my ideal figure would drop from above. In one fell swoop, off would come the saddle bags, the belly fat, the excess flesh under the arms, the double chin. It would be completely painless, and no blood would be shed. Voilà! Perfect me.

But there is no magic cure. It's up to you, and I know you can do it.

You Are Not a Failure

Just because you're the one whose untamed mind is responsible for your counterproductive behaviors doesn't mean you're a failure at reaching your right size. Or that you're weak and undisciplined. Or that you're a horrible person who doesn't deserve to be free of this burden. Are you filled with shame for your shortcomings? I've been there and it is excruciating.

Putting yourself down does not work. I mean, *really*. Has shaming yourself ever changed your behavior? I'm not talking about how others shamed you—that's a different discussion. Think about times that *you shaming yourself* worked for you.

Name one time… I'll wait…

You're not a failure, and you're not a horrible person. You did the best you could, given inadequate tools and your level of awareness and maturity at the time. Meanwhile, there is one more possibility you must consider…

You really do NOT want to lose weight. *Society says* you should lose weight; *your partner says* you should lose weight; *your doctor says* you should lose weight. However, your efforts have been half-hearted at best. Maybe it's time to acknowledge that *you do not want to change.*

I get it; I make an annual New Year's resolution to create a daily meditation practice, and yet I don't follow through. Change requires effort and commitment, and thus far my reasons aren't compelling enough. If that's where you're at right now, congratulations for owning up to the truth!

Would you just as soon forever exit the weight-loss battlefield? Lindy West, author of the memoir *Shrill*, writes about coming to that moment of recognizing she had been fat since birth and would never be a thin person. It infuriated her that fat people are only acceptable if they make a public show of their weight-loss efforts. The hell with that, she decided. She stopped dieting, stopped trying to be someone she isn't, and says she is happy with herself exactly as she is—a fat woman.

So, let's get some clarity here. In this exercise, you're going to play the devil's advocate and explore the possibility that *you do not want to change—you no longer want to lose weight.* (I can already hear you disagreeing, but give this exercise a go anyway.)

Prompt: Why I don't want to lose weight. As a brainstorming exercise in your notebook, list every imaginable reason you might want to keep your weight problem—no reason too absurd—just dump them out without editing or censoring. "I look more approachable as a fat person." "I'm sick of feeling deprived." "If I lose weight, my fat friends won't like me anymore." "My weight keeps sex partners at bay." Your turn. Go…

If you discover from this writing exercise that you would prefer to make peace with your size *as it is*, and no longer want to "try" to lose weight, you can still benefit from using the tools in this book to get more pleasure from your food, so read on.

Taking Responsibility

To take responsibility means acknowledging you made some unskillful choices in the past. It means recognizing that *you and only you* can make more skillful choices going forward. Know this: if you're mindful, you always have a choice to act in the direction of your goals.

***Unless you have specific medical restrictions or an eating disorder,* no foods are off limits here.** Your success will depend on implementing simple practices that will shift how you relate to food and to your body—from enemy to essential allies. These practices will challenge your entrenched habits of eating unconsciously, stuffing your feelings, and believing your well-crafted justifications.

You will do this imperfectly—over and over. Remember when you first learned to walk? You fell frequently. Every time you fell, you got up and tried it again. Pretty soon you were off and running. Equally important, despite frequent falls, you never trash-talked yourself. Be like that baby. The more you practice, the sooner these behaviors will become second nature.

These practices may also change your life. As a former Thin Within participant, Joni K. wrote me, "I've lost 20 pounds in the years since I took the seminar, but more importantly, food is no longer a threat. I hadn't realized how much it ran me. This positive feeling of mastery overflows to my whole life."

• • • • • REMEMBER THIS • • • • •

- You were the one who put the food in your mouth.
- When you accept that you are responsible, you can choose differently.
- Practice + Patience = Progress

5

Calibrating Your Fuel Gauge: SuperTool #1

Don't let your eyes get bigger than your stomach.

—Mom

Before we begin the regular practices that will help you achieve your weight goals, we've got to calibrate our essential instruments.

Calorie, carbohydrate, points counters. Nope. Put these away. We're not counting.

The scales. Nope. Not them either. This instrument is not your friend. It reports too late—well after the deed is done. What you overate yesterday is already on its way to your hips. Here's what happens when you weigh yourself. If your weight registers higher on the scales, you feel terrible about yourself, so you might as well keep eating, since you've already screwed up. Or, let's say you step on the scales and it reports you've *lost* a couple of pounds. *Whoopee!* Now you can eat more. Gain or lose, whenever you weigh yourself, you lose. You've turned your power over to this dumb machine to determine how you should feel about yourself. So, hop on the scale for what I hope is the last time for at least several weeks, and maybe forever. Record the number in your notebook for your starting point, then shove the nasty contraption to the back of the closet.

Your internal fuel gauge. Yes! Now we're talking. Wouldn't it be great to have a built-in fuel gauge? Like in a car, it would always be visible on your mental dashboard to measure how much food was in your tank. However, your car has two additional features: the gas tank cannot expand, no matter how tasty the fuel, and a valve in the nozzle prevents you from topping off.

Since Humans 1.0 still lack fuel gauges or shut-off valves, we have to resort to our inner sensors to tell us: where on the continuum between hunger and fullness are we right now? And now? And now? This sensor, once it's calibrated, will let you know how much is in that **two-pint pot**, better known as the stomach. And it can make or break your success at losing or maintaining weight.

Growing up, my mom often told us not to let our eyes get bigger than our stomachs when we piled our plates unreasonably high. "You can't fit a quart into a pint pot," she'd warn.

In its normal shape, an adult stomach holds about two pints (a quart) of food and liquid. However, the stomach is remarkably elastic and can expand to contain four times that much. That's why we have to loosen our belts toward the end of Thanksgiving dinner. Back in our cave-dwelling days, this elasticity proved lifesaving, because it might be a long time before we caught the next wildebeest.

We won't die if we abstain from alcohol, cigarettes, and other addictive substances. Not so with food; our bodies need fuel to survive. But how much food is *just enough*, and how can you figure out what is the *too much* that bulges your belly or adds another chin?

Am I hungry? When I first gave up dieting, it never occurred to me to ask myself if I was actually hungry. If it was mealtime, I must be hungry, so I ate. If food was put in front of me, I ate. If I knew I'd be out past mealtime, I ate preventively.

Am I full? Furthermore, it never occurred to me to ask myself if I was full. If food remained on the plate, I must still be hungry.

Does this sound familiar?

How Does Hunger Feel? And Where Do We Feel It?

A lot is happening inside our bodies 24/7 that we only notice when we're directed to become aware of what the inner action feels like, as in meditation, or when a sensation is particularly strong (like a full bladder, a racing heart, stomach gas). Awareness of these sensations is called interoception—like perception, but directed internally, not externally. Most of the time our obliviousness to our body's inner workings is no big deal. The brain is making sure all systems are go, regardless of whether we're aware of them. However, certain signals call us into action. Without food, the brain can't function, so awareness of our hunger and fullness sensations is a survival skill.

Physiological hunger is not the same as appetite, which is the desire to eat food regardless of your hunger state. True hunger pangs are stomach contractions that begin to occur between 12 and 24 hours after last eating and are triggered by low nutrient levels in the blood, and by hormonal and nerve signals from the GI tract to the brain.

Most of us who can afford to buy food rarely allow ourselves to experience physiological hunger for more than a couple of hours. We succumb instead to psychological hunger, which doesn't come from the stomach; it resides in the mind. It's triggered when we see food or other people eating, when negative feelings arise (stress, indecision, fatigue, grief, anger, loneliness, shame, etc.), and when we're faced with an unpleasant or confusing task. We also may experience it in the mouth as a desire to chew or suck, or a grabby feeling in the hands to get something to put in the mouth.

Becoming attuned to your body's hunger and fullness signals is a practice that is essential to forging a healthier relationship to your food.

What Does Fullness Feel Like? And Where Do We Feel It?

Satiety is another word for fullness—it's a sensation that we're satisfied by what we've just eaten, and it's determined by a complex mix of physical sensations from the stomach, hormonal signals, and taste buds, as well as our surroundings and emotional state. Foods high in fat, in protein (meat, poultry, fish, beans), in nutrient density (vegetables, fruits, whole grains), and water (soups, stews) tend to make us feel satiated sooner. On the other hand, alcoholic beverages can stimulate the appetite and dull our ability to discern when we're full.

The Okinawans have an expression, *hara hachi bun me*, that reminds them to eat only until their bellies are 80% full. The accompanying proverb, "Eight parts of a full stomach sustain the man; the other two sustain the doctor," seems to be borne out by their renowned longevity. I'm guessing this practice means *stop eating before the stomach stretches*. And if you want to lose weight, stopping before you hit 70% is a good idea.

Language matters. When we describe hunger in the English language, we say, "I am hungry" and "I am full," identifying (equating) ourselves with those sensations. The French say, "J'ai faim," which translates to "I *have* hunger." When the French are full, they say, "Je n'ai plus faim" —"I no longer have hunger" (my hunger is sated). You can see how *being full* is very different from having eaten *just enough*. It's time to stop focusing on whether you're full, and notice instead if you've had just enough.

My own children were more in touch with their fuel level than I was back then. Even as babies, they knew when they'd had enough and made sure I knew. Their tiny teeth clamped down on the spoon, and "Pffft!" out would come the offending bite. Once the mouth shut, it stayed shut—not even opening for my "watch the flying spoon" games.

We can't control the behavior of our satiation hormones, but we can control how much we eat before they kick in and say, "FULL!"

SuperTool #1: Tuning Your Internal Fuel Gauge

If you want to lose weight and keep it off, your internal fuel gauge is key to your success. You'll be relying on it every day for the rest of your life. In short, you'll learn (most of the time) to wait to eat until you're physiologically hungry, and to stop well before you're full—when you've had just enough.

I don't recommend letting your fuel level drop to 0, where you'd eat your leather belt if it wasn't holding up your pants. The sweet spot is the zone between 30% and 70%. Below 20%, your brain is struggling to give you the energy and focus you need to function. Above 80%, you're having to unbutton your waistband to make space and you're becoming increasingly uncomfortable.

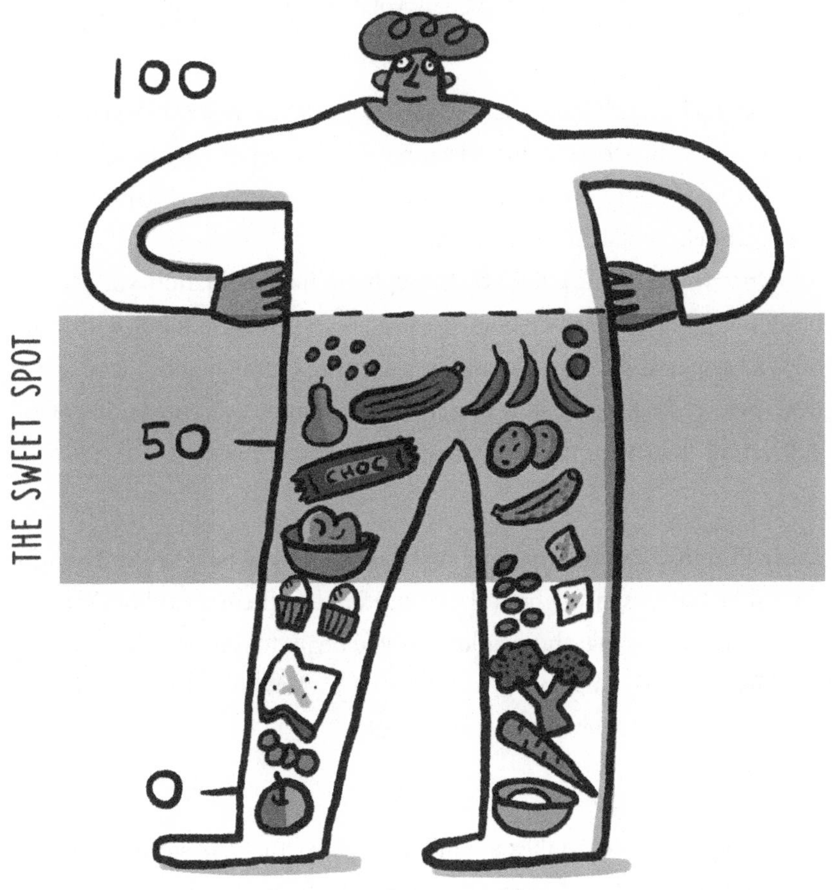

I can't tell you what your fuel levels feel like because each person's sensory data map is unique, but the following exercises will help familiarize you with the various sensations you associate with hunger and fullness at different times of day and during meals. You can then begin to connect certain sensations with each level. With regular practice, your fuel level awareness will become sharper and, eventually, automatic.

Guided Meditation: Discovering Your Internal Fuel Gauge [Listen here: joyoverstreet.com/pie]. Do not skip this essential exercise, where you'll begin to identify your own hunger and fullness sensations. Seat yourself in a straight-back chair and let me guide you through this process.

Your fuel gauge has been ignored so long it may be rusty or even broken; it may take a while to get it up and running. Please repeat the above process of checking your fuel levels several times a day, especially as you think about eating or believe that you're hungry.

Once you've let me guide you through this first meditation, you should be able to guide yourself through the process of getting in touch with your body's hunger and fullness sensations. Getting in touch with these sensations before, during and after you eat is an essential awareness skill you're cultivating. Take your time to notice *in this present moment.*

Daily Practice: Tuning up your fuel gauge. For the next seven days, do several fuel checks throughout the day and record them on a chart like the one below. What's your hunger level as you begin to eat? What and where are those hunger sensations? If your starting level is above 50%, record what else might have triggered that desire to eat.

Because the brain takes a while to register that the stomach is satiated, you will need to sloooow down. Savor the food, chew more, take a deep breath and look around, put your fork down between bites. Drink some water.

As you finish eating, examine your experience of satiation. At what moment do you feel you've had enough? When you're bored with what's on your plate? When the plate is clean? Is it a sensation around your waist or above your waist? What is your hunger level as you finish each eating session? Write these numbers down. Examples:

Hunger Levels at Several Points During the Day

B% = Hunger Level ***Before*** eating **A%** = Hunger Level ***After*** eating

Time	B%	Situation	Sensations/Emotions?	A%	Notes
8:15 a.m.	20%	Breakfast time	Stomach growling	70%	I'm bored of Cheerios
10 a.m.	60%	Passed bowl of Halloween candy on co-worker's desk	Hands want to grab a few	30%	Didn't eat any, but made me feel hungry
3:30 p.m.	50%	Dealing with a cranky child	Tired, fed up	70%	Ate 6 wheat crackers
6:15 p.m.	40%	Dinner time	Mild hunger, offset by glass of wine. Mellow	80%	Full—wine dulled my focus
9 p.m.	70%	Too tired to do anything, but too wired for bed	Heavy eyes, don't feel like moving	90%	Ate bowl of ice cream, why?

You can actually graph your hunger levels during the day. Do this for a couple of weeks and you will begin to discover common patterns. [Reminder: all charts can be found on my website, joyoverstreet.com/pie organized by chapter.]

Graphing Daily Hunger Levels

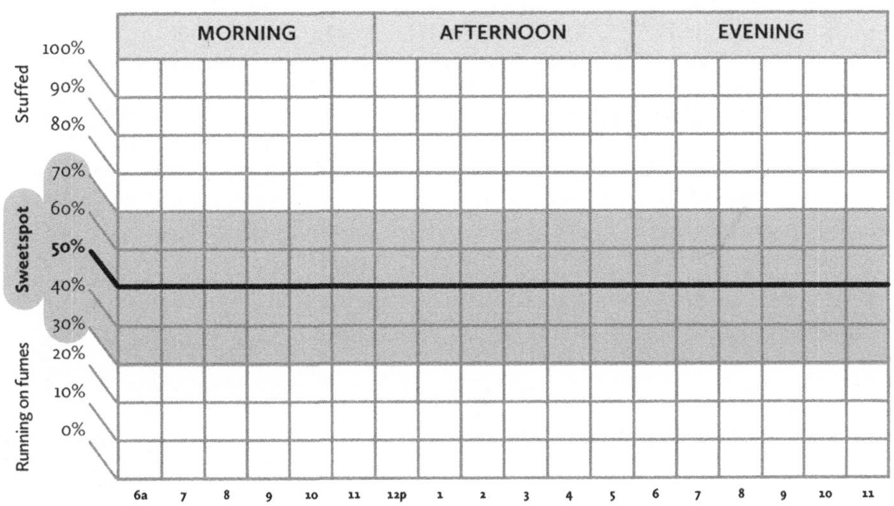

• • • • • REMEMBER THIS • • • • •

- Becoming aware of how unaware you are is the first step in waking up.
- If you want to lose weight:
    - Wait to eat until your tank is below 30%
    - Stop eating before your tank reaches 70%

6

Calibrating Your Eyes

You've got one other instrument that needs calibrating—your eyes.

In the absence of rulers, scales, measuring cups and so forth, we rely on our eyes to gauge the size of something by context—what it's next to. You can eat eight ounces from a gallon of ice cream before it looks like you've made a dent in it, whereas if you eat the same amount from a pint, it would be obvious, because half has disappeared.

During the next two or three weeks, you'll be collecting data on your eating habits by keeping a food diary. You won't need to measure, weigh, or count the calories of anything you eat, but recording what you eat with relative precision is another way to keep yourself honest. (I know how easy it is to call a giant heap "a serving.")

Eating satisfaction is as much mental as it is physical. When we eat off a small plate heaped with food, our eyes suggest we're getting a lot, so we feel satisfied with less than if we were served the same amount on a large one.

In the 1950s, the average dinner plate was 9 inches in diameter. Today it is 11 inches. You'd think an inch or two wouldn't matter much, but it's a question of area, not diameter. A 9-inch plate is 64 square inches; an 11-inch plate is 95 square inches—a surface area 39% greater. Today's 12-inch restaurant plate can accommodate 113 square inches of food. If you search on the internet for "average dinner plate size," you'll see many images of different size plates showing how puny or ample food looks on them. Liquid in a tall, skinny glass looks like more than it does in a short, fat one. A single serving of wine (5 ounces or about 2/3 cup) in a wide-bottomed goblet looks skimpy compared to the same amount in a champagne flute. A narrower glass could be the ticket if you want to drink less without feeling cheated.

Test your eyes. Make a small pot of rice or mashed potatoes or oatmeal (something that hangs together fairly well) and scoop some into a one-cup measure, some into a half-cup measure, and some into a quarter-cup measure. Place a one-cup scoop onto your usual dinner plate. Notice how much space the scoop occupies, and how much open space surrounds it on the plate. Now move the scoop to a salad plate. Again, notice how much space it takes and how much open space is left. Repeat this process with each of the other two scoops.

You'll need to consider other measurements as well. When is a "sip" really a big gulp? How many ounces are in your glass of wine or your soft drink? When is a "bite" half of the cookie? What percent of a piece of pie or toast is "crust?" Is "half a bag of chips" a mega-bag or snack-size? You get the idea. I know all the sleazy tricks we play on ourselves. Aim for honesty.

• • • • • REMEMBER THIS • • • • •

- Our perception of quantity is relative.
- Your eyes often trick your stomach.

PART TWO

Start Where You Are

You can't assess your progress unless you know your starting point. What's true right now? Are you as aware of your eating patterns as you thought? Are you and your body friends or enemies? As a self-scientist, you begin to collect the important data you'll need for this voyage of discovery.

7

Square One

"Start where you are," is great advice *if* you know where that is. Too often, our perspective on an emotionally charged area of our lives is warped. As therapist Lori Gottlieb says, "Part of getting to know yourself is to unknow yourself—to let go of the limiting stories you've told yourself about who you are so that you aren't trapped by them."

I hope you've filled out the "Before" questionnaire in Appendix A, so you've begun to pinpoint your current situation, the history of your weight struggles, and the state of the rest of your life. I asked a bunch of questions about what's going on in the rest of your life because it is all connected.

For example, my mind was so engulfed by my weight worries that I had little energy available for much else, like my kids. Some nights I could barely sleep, and other nights ten hours in bed wasn't enough. In the first month after my Cherry Pie Epiphany, my sleep leveled out and my energy soared. Just recognizing that I was on the right path diminished my obsession with those extra pounds and made me a much more present parent. When you do the "After" questionnaire some weeks or months from now, you'll be able to compare what has shifted.

Your "Fat Story"

This origin story is an important aspect of your starting point. It's your best understanding of how your weight problem emerged and what seems to be holding it in place. Because this narrative still runs its subversive tape in some dark corner of your brain, it can affect who you think you are and how you behave around food. Once it's out in the open, the sunlight begins to bleach out the fear and shame.

Many find it hard to believe someone as slim and omnivorous as I've been for the last four decades ever struggled. I have photos to prove it. Here's my tale.

Joy's Fat Story

Back in 1956, my parents wanted a vacation from kids, so they shipped us off to Camp Wyonegonic in Maine for two months. Even though I was fifteen and old enough to keep myself amused all summer at home, my folks were sick of my sullen, surly, boy-crazy presence. In retrospect, I can't say I blame them.

I considered myself way too cool for camp, plus I hated anything athletic. My favorite "sport" was climbing our old maple tree to sit among the branches with a book. But off I went, determined to be miserable, just to show them.

I was homesick, lonely, and angry. In those eight weeks, I did pull off one impressive accomplishment: I gained 25 pounds—an average of more than 3 pounds per week.

Under my parents' roof, staying slim required little thought. My mother prepared healthy meals, much of it from our own large garden. She rarely served desserts and soda pop was forbidden. (Only many years later did I recognize how fortunate we were not to get habituated to sweets as kids.)

In contrast, camp food was, well, camp food—fatty, rich, sweet, and very ample. The extra physical activity was no match for the calories on the table, which I wolfed down without a second thought. I drowned my meatloaf in gravy, my bologna sandwiches in mayonnaise, the iceberg wedges in Russian dressing. I developed a real thing for potato chips, to the point where I crumbled them on the well-dressed iceberg wedges, on soup, and for crunch, stuck into the middle of my sandwiches. Best of all—real dessert after lunch ***and*** dinner!

To me, every meal was a happy meal. I ate ***everything***, oblivious to the increasing tightness of my camp uniform. Hence, at the end of August when Mom picked us up at the train station, I was as surprised by her shocked expression (***what's she looking at?***) as she was shocked by the inflated version of the daughter she'd left at the station two months earlier.

Her eyes widened. She blinked a few times and finally exclaimed, "Mmmm-boy! Are you... uh... er... uh... ***healthy***!"

Then I knew. We were big fans of comedian Jackie Gleason's TV show, and she had just stopped herself from delivering one of his favorite lines: "Mmmm-boy! Are you FAT!" I looked down at my chunky legs. I felt my belly pushing on the waistband of my shorts.

She was right. I hated her for noticing, and I hated ***her*** because my fat was TOTALLY HER FAULT for sending me away.

It got worse. At the first school dance of the year, Jack Patterson, the senior boy I had an enormous crush on, asked me to dance. I floated twice around the floor in his arms, until one of his buddies called out to him, "Hey Jack! What's it like to dance with a Mack truck?"

My face flamed. He was talking about ***me***. I fled the dance in shame.

I would have to go on a diet, but what? Some of my girlfriends swore by Metrecal, the chalky, glurpy precursor to SlimFast. It tasted disgusting. However, in its favor was the self-limiting nature of the little can. What if I brought a little can of something else? I chose LeSeuer's Super Sweet Fancy Tiny Peas, a food I loved. At first. Nevertheless, I doggedly stuck to my Pea Diet most of the fall, although my friends teased me without mercy.

By Christmas I'd lost the 25 pounds. It never occurred to me that a return to my mom's nutritious meals might have been the decisive factor rather than my Pea Diet. However, from then on I became an inveterate diet dabbler, believing that only a diet and constant vigilance would keep me slim.

I was wrong.

And that's where we circle back to my pity party on the couch in 1975, when I gave up dieting for good.

✏📖 **Prompt: Write your "Fat Story."** It's your turn to get your narrative on paper so you can begin to put it behind you. As you write, give the story all the dramatic flourishes it deserves. What happened first? And then what? Is there a villain in this tale (someone besides yourself)? After you've finished writing it down, read it aloud to yourself. Are there parts that still hurt? Are there parts that in retrospect seem overblown or even silly? Are there parts that another witness to the tale would have described differently? Make some notes about your story from the perspective you have today. Can you allow your current self to move on?

Beware the Unreliable Narrator

The protagonist in fiction (and the client in therapy work) is often what's called an "unreliable narrator." This means the storyteller shapes the tale to serve their own purposes, editing out certain details and embellishing others. Now, take a look back at the third paragraph of my fat story where I describe myself as homesick, lonely, and angry—implying that my miseries caused my overeating.

Well. It just so happens…

Very recently I cleaned out a file box of memorabilia from my youth and came across a letter to my parents from the director of Camp Wyonegonic, reporting how my two sisters and I were faring at mid-summer. By the director's account, I had lots of friends, enjoyed many camp activities, and had taken a leadership role in some of them. I was stunned.

I would have dismissed the director's observations as trying to assure my parents they'd made a wise choice in sending me to camp, except she said of my middle sister, "She does not like it here, and I think she would be very happy not to return next year."

Was I that skillful in hiding my misery? Or had I added the misery detail way back then so I could blame my mother for my wanton face-stuffing? I suspect the latter. My mother was a favorite scapegoat for my sins.

As you look back at your own "fat story," can you imagine that you might have sculpted some of the narrative's details for your own purposes? These stories shape our identities in powerful ways, as therapist Lori Gottlieb describes so well in her TEDTalk, and her book, *Maybe You Should Talk to Someone*. Change your story/identity, change your life. We'll get there in Parts Three and Four.

REMEMBER THIS

- Your fat story is not your destiny.
- Your fat story may not even be true.
- A fresh story begins in the present moment.

8

Is Anybody Home When You Eat?

The truth will set you free,
but first it will piss you off.
—Twelve Step aphorism

I know that you believe you're present when you eat. I certainly believed I was—I mean, I love food, love to eat, why wouldn't I be present to enjoy it? And yet, too often I'd look down at my empty plate (or bowl or carton or bag), only to realize I had no idea where the food had gone.

Here's your chance to assess your default eating mode by following a guided meditation—a reality show we'll call ***Me: Eating.*** The exercise is much more effective if you can listen to the meditation instead of trying to read and imagine at the same time.

Guided Meditation: "Me, Eating" [Reminder: all meditations are available for listening at my website's private page, joyoverstreet.com/pie.]

To prepare for this unique performance, set aside 15 minutes and find a comfy place to sit where nobody will disturb you. Close your eyes and let your imagination build the story. There is no right or wrong way to do this, no particular images you're supposed to see. Take whatever you get.

Prompt: "Me, Eating" meditation takeaways. Spend a few minutes writing in your notebook what you noticed during the meditation. In each situation, what enhanced your eating experience? What detracted from it? Were you able to focus on your food or were you distracted by thoughts, the situation? Did you eat more than you intended? Did you eat anything you didn't really like? Did you finish everything? Did you notice any emotions during this meal? If you could have a do-over, how would you script it? Add any additional thoughts, memories, or judgments the meditation may have sparked.

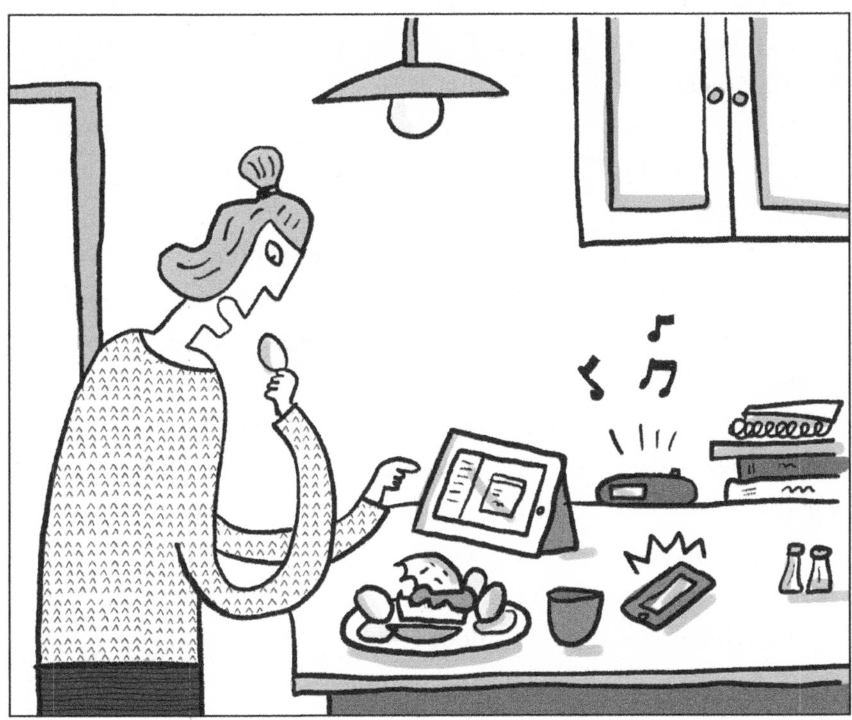

9

You Have a Body

You have a body. Without your body, the person everyone knows as You wouldn't exist. The body is something we have in common with every other living being. It's the sensing organ that connects us to each other and to all experience. When you get right down to it, your body is so profoundly important that it's ridiculous not to treat it with reverence, as the gift that it is—whatever its condition—to relish its quirks and to nurture it with love. As the late yoga master B.K.S. Iyengar said, "It is through your body that you realize you are a spark of divinity."

Right now your body doesn't meet your exacting standards. It's not the shape that celebrity magazines put on their cover. It suffers from twinges, bulges, sags, aches, colds and coughs, wrinkles and zits. It may even have an illness that will kill it.

When you live inside enemy territory, it's difficult to be happy.

From the time I was an adolescent until my Thin Within experience, I had a body that never pleased me. It was too flat-chested; it had saddle-bag thighs and turkey-neck upper arms; it felt weak and clumsy; and at times it weighed between 12 and 25 pounds too much. My body got stuffed with too much food—foods I knew were bad for it and foods I didn't even like. And then I blamed my body when the crunchy peanut butter ended up around my waist.

Decades ago, my friend Chérie Carter-Scott created a list she called "Ten Rules for Being Human," later immortalized by Jack Canfield in *Chicken Soup for the Soul.* Eventually Chérie expanded her list into a bestselling book, *If Life is a Game, These are the Rules: Ten Rules for Being Human*. Here's the first rule:

> ***Rule One.*** *You will receive a body. You may love it or hate it, but it will be yours for the duration of your life on Earth.*
>
> *The moment you arrived here on this Earth, you were given a body in which to house your spiritual essence. The real "you" is stored inside this body—all the hopes, dreams, fears, thoughts, expectations and beliefs that make you the unique human that you are...*
>
> *Since there is a no-refund, no-exchange policy on this body of yours, it is essential that you learn to transform your body from a mere vessel into a beloved partner and lifelong ally, as the relationship between you and your body is the most fundamental and important relationship of your lifetime. It is the blueprint from which all your other relationships will be built...*
>
> *The challenge of Rule One is to make peace with your body, so that it can effectively serve its purpose and share its valuable lessons of acceptance, self-esteem, respect, and pleasure.*

Since my body was the vehicle for all I could be or do in this life, I knew I'd have to make friends with it. I set off on an acceptance mission. My first step was to acknowledge that the body I inhabited was mine, my one and only vehicle, in "as is" condition—to have and to hold, for better or for worse, in sickness and in health, as long as we both shall live.

We get out of touch with our own bodies for many reasons, including:

- We live in our heads
- We want to deny our size
- We want to deny our sexuality

- We compare ourselves unfavorably to others
- We carry emotional pain from the past
- We are ashamed to be who we (think we) are

You cannot exist without your body. So, isn't it time to begin building a kinder, more compassionate relationship to it?

We'll start with a meditative exploration of the body you have right now.

Standing Body Meditation: Remove your shoes if you're wearing heels and put down anything you might have in your hands. Find a place in the room where you can stand without being concerned about bumping into something when your eyes are shut. (If standing is a problem, you can also do this in a straight-back chair.) Stand with your feet slightly apart, and rock back and forth until you feel well-grounded. Start the meditation audio, and then close your eyes.

Prompt: When I feel my body... At the end of the meditation, take out your notebook and jot down what you noticed as you brought awareness to each part of your body. Any surprises? Emotions?

You can return to this exercise at any time to get back in touch with your body.

"Advanced" Standing Body Meditation. Stand naked in front of a full-length mirror, with your eyes open, and repeat the meditation above. Please, please, please—talk to your various body parts in a kind and compassionate way. Acknowledge that shaming voice and tell it to keep its damned opinions to itself.

REMEMBER THIS

- It's hard to be happy if you live inside enemy territory.
- Your body is not a rental car. It's for keeps.
- Would you treat your dearest friend the way you treat your body?

10

The Data Doesn't Lie: SuperTool #2

What ails the truth is that it is mainly uncomfortable, and often dull. The human mind seeks something more amusing, and more caressing. Into our most solemn and serious reflections fictions enter and three times out of four they quickly crowd out the facts.

—H.L. Mencken

The painful truth was that I had been eating more than my body burned, mostly without me even noticing. After deciding to quit dieting forever, the very first thing I did was to keep track of what I was putting in my mouth, because I knew in my dark little heart that I had been using magical thinking when it came to how much I was eating.

I pretended that eating my kids' crusts didn't count. Taste testing the stew I was making didn't count, nor did licking the brownie batter off the spoon. Making the edges even on the leftover casserole didn't count. The potato chips that fell to the floor by the coffee table didn't count either.

Although many diets had asked me to track and count calories or carbohydrates, I felt it was beneath my dignity, so I never did it. As a newly minted self-scientist, however, I recognized the need for a collection of accurate data. What *was* I putting in my mouth throughout the day? Not just *what,* but when, where, how much, and why? Only with that information would I be able to figure out what changes were called for.

I started with a simple food diary, just recording six data points each time I ate something: time of day, location, hunger levels before and after, name of food, approximation of the amount. No amount was too tiny to escape recording. A bite here. A crust there. A lick. A smidge. A crumb. I forced myself not to change my customary behavior, because as soon as I started writing down all those bites-that-don't-count, an embarrassing pattern began to emerge. I ate like a cow (minus the extra stomachs), grazing all day long.

Super Tool #2 Accurate Data Collection

You may have kept food diaries before, and hated it. I agree; it's super annoying. You will want to cheat. You will want to change your behavior so you don't have to write it down. But this is information you're going to need in order to see where the glitches are. Recording what you eat, *as you're eating it*, without trying to "look good," helps you become aware of what you're doing. For the moment, continue to clean up the cake crumbs and broken chips and record them all. As you review the data in your notebook at the end of the day, and at the end of each week, you'll begin to see patterns in your food choices, eating habits, hunger levels, emotional states, pleasure (or lack of it), and so much more. Soon enough you'll choose to ignore the broken cookie.

Fortunately, it will only take a couple of weeks to amass most of the data you need. You won't need to measure, weigh, or count the calories, carbohydrates, or points of anything you eat, but you do need to tell the truth as you write it down. "Just a serving" is too often one of the lies we tell ourselves. This is why I asked you to make those test piles of mashed potatoes in chapter 5, so you know roughly how a half cup or cup looks on your plate.

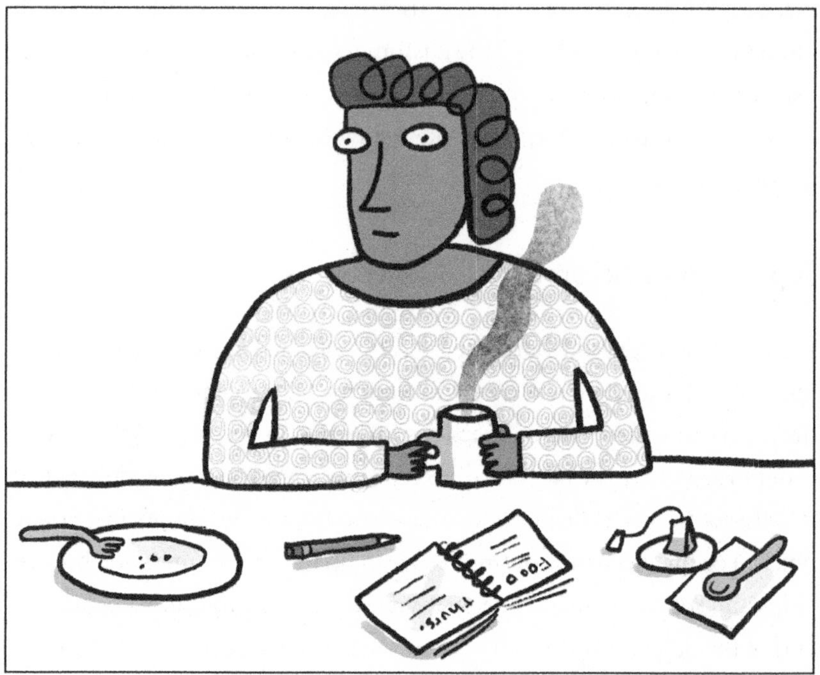

Practice: The food diary—week one. In your notebook, make a chart for recording your food intake. This is where you'll write down every single thing you eat and drink, noting time and place. Yes, even include crumbs from straightening the edge of the cake. Note your hunger level (%) when you begin eating and when you stop. The sample format is below.

Do this every day for seven days, while you're eating. Attempting to reconstruct this information at bedtime *does not work.*

At the end of the day, review your food diary and summarize any patterns you notice. Also make note of particular foods you enjoyed, and those that bored you. At the end of the week, look back at the entire week and write about what stands out.

My Truthful Food Diary, Day, Date ____________

B% = Hunger Level ***Before*** eating **A%** = Hunger Level ***After*** eating

Time	B%	Place	Food/Amount	A%

Observations at the end of the day:

You've got your reasons. For the second week of data collecting, you'll be adding one more column to your food diary: **Why I ate this.** All too often, we eat for reasons that have nothing to do with hunger. We tell ourselves little stories about the food—sometimes these are merely running commentary and sometimes they are justifications for eating when we're not hungry or don't like the food.

Practice: The Food Diary—Week Two. Why I ate this. As you eat, for each item on your list give your reason for eating that particular thing. Do this for seven days, while you're eating.

My Truthful Food Diary, with Reasons **Day, Date** ____________

B% = Hunger Level ***Before*** eating **A%** = Hunger Level ***After*** eating

Time	B%	Food/Amount	A%	Why I ate this

Observations at the end of the day:

When I did this exercise, I discovered my most frequent reason was simply, "It was there." Here are some other favorites:

- I'm bored.
- I'm confused—unsure what to do right now.
- I'm too stressed to think.
- It's six o'clock.
- I love mashed potatoes!
- I need fuel to keep going.
- I don't want to do what I know needs doing.

- Hmmm… Is that as tasty/interesting as it looks?
- It's just a *teeny* piece.
- Salad/kale/broccoli is good for me.
- It's too much work to wrap it and put it in the fridge.
- I already ate something I shouldn't have, so I might as well keep eating.
- *Just in case…* I might get hungry while I'm out.
- I need to show my kids that it's edible/not too hot/cold/spicy/whatever.
- My host would think I'm rude if I didn't eat it.
- I *deserve* it.

At the end of week two, review your food diary for all seven days. What stands out? Did any of your "reasons" actually produce your desired result?

✏📖 **Prompt: Make a list of your reasons for eating.** Create a page in your notebook where you list the reasons you noted in your food diary. You can add to it as your mind coughs them up over the next few weeks. What are your three most frequent reasons? Which ones seem "valid" and which seem flimsy or downright bogus on closer inspection?

• • • • • REMEMBER THIS • • • • •

- We eat for a hundred reasons besides the body's need for fuel.
- Many of your reasons are bogus.
- Feeding your unpleasant feelings only postpones the inevitable.

11

The Winning Formula: SuperTool #3

You must be present to win.
—Raffle ticket stub

I know you were thrilled to toss your calorie and carb counters, your lists of what you could and couldn't eat. Whoopee! No more rules! Well, almost. The prerequisite for losing weight without dieting is ***consciousness***. You must be *present* to win—or if you want to lose that extra weight.

You may have noticed in the **"Me: Eating"** meditation that you weren't as present as you could have been, or that the situation wasn't conducive to being mindful. It's OK. Our Thin Within participants always groaned in dismay when they mentally replayed their meals.

To lose or maintain your weight, while enjoying your food more than ever, AND never again resorting to a diet, three conditions must be in place.

1. **You must be able to focus on eating when you eat.** That means you're sitting down, in a relatively calm environment, at a place set up for eating. It means you are not distracted by the TV, your cell phone, a magazine, your to-do lists. It means you take a few deep breaths to center yourself and let go of other concerns, at least for a few minutes. Here is my favorite centering mantra from my friend Veronika Noize:

   Breathing in I calm my body; breathing out my doubt and fear

   Breathing in deep relaxation; breathing out, my mind is clear

   Breathing in this grateful moment; I am fully present here.

When you focus on what you're eating, you won't suffer the embarrassing experience of looking down at an empty plate, unaware of what you ate or how it disappeared. If you're eating with others, alternate between eating a few bites and (*fork down*) attending to the conversation.

2. **You must pay attention to the signals from your body—your internal fuel gauge.** Put SuperTool #1 into practice. Are you actually hungry (at 30% or less), or are you eating for other reasons? Your appetite or your food may not coincide with your usual meal times. Ask yourself, "Am I actually hungry, or do I just want to change how I feel?" When in doubt, *don't eat.* You will not starve, and you may learn something important about what emotional discomfort you're trying to avoid.

   Are you eating slowly enough that your fuel gauge has time to register? As the meal or snack progresses, how much empty space do you still have inside? Have you eaten just enough to be sated (no more than 70% full), or are you eating until the food is gone? When in doubt, break the automatic hand-to-mouth spell by putting your fork/spoon/hand down and leaving the table briefly for a glass of water or a visit to the bathroom. You can also take your plate to the sink, so it's out of tempting sight range.

3. **You must use all your senses to experience *what* you're eating—in the present moment.** How does the food look? How does it feel and sound in your mouth? Smell and taste? Is the fifth bite as good as the first? Do you like the food? What is it about each item that appeals to you—the salty, spicy, sweet, crunchy, the mouth feel? Is any part of it unappealing? If you routinely make these observations, you'll become a much more discriminating eater, and quite possibly a better cook as well.

   If you don't like the food, can you leave it uneaten? Face it, you'll never be able to eat *everything*, so you might as well enjoy what you *are* eating. Furthermore, your mother isn't watching. Why waste precious calories on food you don't like? It will only bulge your belly.

Winning at Losing

Let me introduce you now to SuperTool #3, the "Winning Formula," the essential set of guidelines you'll be using to reach and stay at your weight goal. These "optimum conditions for conscious eating," as we used to call them, are designed to keep you in the present moment with your body and the food before you. This way, the choices you make (to eat or not to eat, to taste or not to taste) are intentional. You can use the Winning Formula regardless of the kind of cuisine you prefer (Cajun, vegan, kosher, *halal*, gluten-free—whatever).

The Winning Formula is simple, but it's also challenging. I promise your unruly mind will want to wander as you sit down to eat—especially when it thinks you're doing something you shouldn't, like eating something "fattening." You will lose track. You will notice you've lost track. Then you'll bring your mind back to your plate and your body. Next, you'll reach for your cell phone or something to read. And once again you will bring your mind back.

Like any new skill, this is challenging at first and requires effort; however, the more you practice, the easier it gets. Here is the good news from current neuroscience. The amazing human brain continues to rewire and reshape itself throughout our lives, based on our repeated behaviors. Eventually, paying attention when you eat will become second nature.

The rewards for using the Winning Formula are many: your taste buds will become more discriminating; you'll get more pleasure from every bite; your body won't feel like a bloated stone at the end of a meal; and you will become leaner and healthier. Most important, these good habits are sustainable to the end of your days.

Remember my mother, the "human garbage pail" in chapter 3? On one of her rare visits to California from New England, she attended the Thin Within class when I introduced the Winning Formula. A few months later, I got a letter from her:

> *You're not going to believe this, but I've lost those pesky 15 pounds I've been carrying since you were born. So many stupid diets! This time all I did was follow those rules you gave me. When you talked about the Clean Plate Club, I realized, uh-oh—that's me! Why do I need to finish every bite? I have a choice. That food could either go to waste, or to my waist.*

Those pounds stayed gone the rest of her long life.

SuperTool #3: The Winning Formula

1. WAIT until you're hungry to eat—internal fuel gauge at 30% or below.
2. Take three deep breaths to center yourself before you eat. If you cannot relax enough to be present to your food and body, WAIT.
3. Sit down at a place set up for eating—not in your car, at your desk or on the couch.
4. Reduce distractions. No TV, radio, reading, or cell phone while you eat.
5. Slow down, so you can stay in communication with your internal fuel gauge.
6. Become aware of the sensory experience of eating the food.
7. If a food doesn't appeal to you, *don't eat it.*
8. STOP eating *before* you're full. Filling up to 70% on your inner fuel gauge is plenty.

The Five-Point Quick Check is an even simpler way to stay conscious as you eat. Begin and end eating with a gut check of your fuel level. In between, do a place, head, and mouth check—touching each spot as you do the check. Making physical gestures helps you to internalize the routine.

The Five-Point Quick Check (Touch each one, in order.)

GUT	Am I actually hungry? (Less than 30%)
PLACE	Am I sitting at a table in a calm environment?
HEAD	Am I centered and able to focus on eating?
MOUTH	Do I taste this food? Do I like it?
GUT	Have I had *just enough*? (No more than 70% full)

Make and post copies of the Winning Formula, then follow it. Tack up these rules wherever you're tempted to eat, like on the refrigerator door, in your car, at your desk. They should burn themselves into your brain.

Once you begin using the Winning Formula as a daily practice, you will see the pounds drop, and your eating pleasure increase. Depending on your goals, you may adjust the fuel gauge percentage that you use to begin or finish eating. Faster weight loss? Wait a bit longer before eating and stop eating sooner. Maintenance? You have more leeway in when to stop eating.

Practice: The Winning Formula Daily Checklist. To keep track of how you're doing with each of the rules, make several copies of the weekly checklist, which you'll see below, as well as in Appendix A, and on my website.

As you go through the day, make a check in each box when you follow that particular rule. Because you will no doubt eat several times each day, each box may have several checks in it.

The Winning Formula Daily Checklist

The Winning Formula Daily Checklist

Make a check mark every time you follow that rule.
Each box can have several checks since you eat several times a day.
At the end of the week look over the chart to see if you notice
any patterns and record your observations.

The Winning Formula	Sun	Mon	Tues	Wed	Thurs	Fri	Sat
1 Wait till you're hungry to eat (fuel gauge at 30% or less)							
2 Take three breaths to center yourself							
3 Sit at a place set up for eating							
4 Reduce distractions (no TV, radio, cell phone, reading)							
5 Slow down and pay attention to your fuel gauge							
6 Be aware of all five senses as you eat							
7 If a food doesn't appeal to you, don't eat it							
8 Stop eating before you're full (fuel gauge at 70%)							

Observations:

• • • • • REMEMBER THIS • • • • •

- Only eat when you're actually hungry.
- Always stop before you're full.
- Savor every bite.

PART THREE

The Enemy in Your Head

· · · · · · · ·

It's time to dig into the many counterproductive ways you've been dealing with your weight—those habitual thinking and behavior patterns that have kept you from succeeding.

This discovery process acts on two levels of awareness—one is sensory (stomach and mouth) and one is in the mind, below ordinary consciousness.

We view reality thru the filter of who we think we are. Each of us constructs our unique identity out of many parts: our genetic makeup; the particular place, time and culture in which we find ourselves; our life experiences; and the stories we tell ourselves to make sense of it all. ("Stories" include your beliefs, assumptions, attitudes, justifications, decisions, amplifications and minimizations.)

Before you can eliminate your inner saboteurs you have to observe them in action. Once they're visible you can make better choices. So drop the shame, please. Instead, as you uncover them try, "Well, now... *that* is interesting!"

12

Negativity Bias

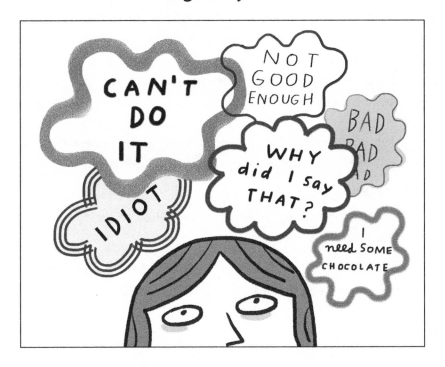

We're multifaceted beings; we have the capacity to hold a variety of self-concepts within us, both positive and negative. The mind wants to make sure we know how we're doing at every given moment, so it keeps up a running commentary—approving and disapproving every move. Unfortunately, the human brain seems to be hard-wired to focus more on our shortcomings. Or, as psychologist Rick Hanson says in his book, *Buddha's Brain*, "Your brain is like Velcro for negative experiences and Teflon for positive ones."

In terms of survival of the species, this makes evolutionary sense. You only stick your hand in the fire once. Poking the bear gets you mauled. Insulting your boss gets you fired. Falling off your diet leads to regaining weight. If we don't learn from negative experiences, we may not survive.

This kind of thinking is called *negativity bias*. While it's useful in keeping us from repeating dangerous behaviors, it's a hindrance in shaping new positive behaviors. The best defense against negativity bias is to recognize it, give it warm thanks for trying to keep you safe, and then tell it to *bug off*.

You may know the parable of the Cherokee chief who was teaching his grandson about life.

> "A fight is going on inside me," he told the young boy, "a fight between two wolves. One is evil and angry. The other is good and peaceful."
>
> The boy looked on, wide-eyed.
>
> "This same fight is going on inside of you, grandson, and inside every other person on this Earth."
>
> The boy pondered this, then asked, "Grandfather, which wolf will win?"
>
> The old man smiled and simply said, "The one you feed."

When I first heard this story, right away I identified one wolf as "fat-mindset" and the other "goal-mindset." (Remember, in this book "fat" is a mental construct, not a particular weight.) It's time to let fat-mindset starve for lack of attention and turn the focus on feeding your goal-mindset.

Fat-mindset keeps the focus on negativity. Your mind says, *You've failed before so you'll probably screw up again. Who are you to think you can succeed this time?* So, you turn to an outside authority, like another diet, hoping for a rescue.

As you will become increasingly aware, the biggest barrier to reaching your sustainable weight goal is all that *blah blah blah* in your head. If you think you're a "fat" person *no matter what you weigh*, you'll never be able to relax around food. You'll never feel good about the body you actually have.

It's a question of identity. *Who you think you are, and who you think you are* not, makes all the difference, because your actions and eating patterns follow who you think you are. This is a core thesis of *The Cherry Pie Paradox*. When you no longer identify as a "fat" person in your mind, you act and eat differently.

So, instead of feeling bad about yourself and all the ways you've "failed" to manage your weight, put down the whip and engage your curiosity. You need to recognize it when you observe it in yourself, so let's explore: what do fat-mindset and fat-behavior look like?

✎📖 **Prompt: How does a person with fat-mindset behave?** Bring to mind someone you know well who struggles with their weight. How do they talk about their body, their diets, or exercise programs? What foods do they eat (at least what you *see*—who knows what happens inside their heads or when they're alone)? What do they appear to avoid? Do they say one thing (about eating) but do something else? Do they blame other people or situations for their behavior? Are they happy with the way they are, or are they hard on themselves? If you've known them for a long time, have you noticed patterns or familiar stories they tell about their weight problems? Do *you* have any evaluations or judgments about them because of their weight?

Repeat this exercise with at least two more people. People who struggle with their weight are as unique as any other humans. The more data you have, the broader your perspective can be.

✎📖 **Prompt:** Write up your notes, then compare them with your own attitudes and behaviors. Mark any similarities to your own with a ✓ and add any others that come to mind. Please, no shame or judgments here! You're just a curious scientist gathering data.

REMEMBER THIS

- To counteract your negativity bias, you first must become aware of your attraction to it.
- Fat-mindset keeps the focus on your fears and failures.
- Thank your fat-mindset for trying to keep you safe. Then tell it to bug off.

13

Don't Call Me a Machine!

Although this occurred in 1973 at the ***est*** training, a popular human potential program of the 1970s and 1980s, I still remember how insulted I felt when the leader, Werner Erhard, called those of us in my group "machines." Some of us argued back. Then he read his definition. "Machine: A constructed thing; one who responds to stimuli without intelligence." He went on: "Machinery: The means by which something is kept in action; the system of organized activities that perpetuates or carries on a process."

He was talking about our habits and thought patterns, which have an automaticity reminiscent of machinery. Definitely no thinking involved. Haven't we all gotten in the car to go to the supermarket and instead find ourselves in the office parking lot? Or bought popcorn every time we go to the movie theater, even though we know it will be terrible?

But: mechanical behavior *can* be helpful. Riding a bike, which originally took all your focus, became second nature with practice. You can make your morning coffee or tie your shoelaces half asleep. The brain likes it when you practice something often enough that it can relax and focus on tasks that require more of its attention, like learning something new.

Still, no one wants to think of themself as a machine, *responding to stimuli without intelligence*, even though we often behave that way around food. I know I did. Much of my eating behavior was so automatic, I came to call it my *fat machinery*.

Three sources of the "machinery" that underlies and perpetuates our counter-productive behaviors:

1. **Past experiences that led to a decision.** At various points in our lives, especially in childhood, we have experiences (positive or negative) that lead us to conclude, ***If X happens, and I do Y, then Z will follow.*** Although your situation may be different today, mere similarity to the prior experience triggers an automatic response. For example, whenever you were in a bad mood, your mom gave you a Hershey's kiss, so you associate chocolate with relief. And now chocolate is your go-to solution for a bad mood. Or you lost lots of weight and yet you still weren't chosen for the cheerleading squad or by the hot date. Since losing weight didn't get you what you wanted, you stopped trying. Of course, these decisions are made way below the level of awareness, otherwise you'd realize they make no sense and act more appropriately.
2. **Habitual responses. A habit is an acquired mode of behavior that has become involuntary.** Originally *habit* referred to a costume one put on, like a nun's habit. Fortunately, if it can be put on, it can also be removed. Some habits are helpful (always putting my keys in the same drawer by the door). Some are weird but innocuous (tying my shoelaces a very peculiar way because I taught myself and am too stubborn to change). Some kept me stuck (opening the refrigerator door whenever I went through the kitchen—then popping a morsel into my mouth).
3. **Beliefs.** A belief is a conviction or assumption that certain things are true, real, or trustworthy. Once we believe something to be true, we don't stop to reexamine it in light of our present experience. **Beliefs filter our reality, like a veil**—so close to the face that we're unaware that what we understand about the world and ourselves has been colored by these filters. A huge proportion of our beliefs are absorbed unconsciously from our families of origin, friends, and the surrounding culture.

When you're a kid, your world is circumscribed. You know little beyond what you experience at home and school. Painful experiences from childhood have an outsized influence (often for life), because your shortened time scale makes the incident proportionally more significant. You're too young to know better, so you assume that *you* must have done something wrong to cause what happened. Only when you get older and meet different kinds of people, encounter other perspectives, and have new experiences, do you begin to question what you believed to be true as a kid. You don't even have to go far from home to get your worldview shaken up, as happened at my breakfast with Carol.

Food and eating have been central (essential!) to our lives since birth, giving us countless opportunities to develop beliefs about them. If weight has been an issue, we've got beliefs about that too. Based on shaming messages of the kind I read in Dr. Rubin's book, I believed that being overweight was a sign of weakness or worse, a moral failing.

Our beliefs don't need to have deep psychological meaning to affect our behavior. For example, in my world, eggs came in pairs and sandwiches had two halves. Because of my unexamined assumptions, it never occurred to me to cook *one* egg or make just *half* a sandwich.

Other common food-related beliefs include: "If it's chocolate it must be delicious;" "You can only lose weight if you cut out carbs;" "Cottage cheese makes you thin;" "It's impossible to eat just one chip;" "Men leave me when I'm thin;" and "A good mother has some padding on her."

It's human nature to want to be *right*, so our beliefs often become self-fulfilling prophecies. As Richard Bach wrote in his bestselling fable, *Jonathan Livingston Seagull*, "Argue for your limitations, and sure enough, they're yours."

Confirmation bias. Often, we try to maintain a particular belief, despite mounting evidence to the contrary. You see this most blatantly in our political views. Whichever way you lean, you tend to follow news sources that confirm what you believe. If a news outlet leans opposite to your views, you won't even bother to check it out. Thanks to your filter, you're only exposed to your preferred reality. And you get to be right. Whoopee.

Let's say you believe overweight people can't (or shouldn't) dance. Instead of noticing that many have a good time dancing and do it very well (which would contradict your bias), you decide you won't even try, even though you would *love* to learn to move like that. By *not* dancing, you don't have the chance to practice moving like that, so guess what? You still don't dance well. So you're right. Again.

We can't see our own beliefs by *thinking* about them. Remember, they veil our perception. How then can we bring these unconscious influences from the past into the light of the present moment so we can make informed choices? The clues are in observing our actions—how we actually conduct our daily lives—like what a video camera would record. We observe our *behavior* with the curiosity of a scientist or a detective. We begin to question. Wait a minute: how come I did that? How come I think that? Is this true? How do I know it's true? Is this belief or behavior still working for me or not? Keep or toss? No judgment, just *curiosity*. Always curiosity.

✎📖 **Prompt: Examine your food diary for beliefs.** Get out your notebook and look over what you ate in the past few days. As you run down the list, see if you can discover any beliefs or preconceptions that led you to choose particular foods. Some foods will be there because you believe them to be "healthy," others because you hoped they'd squash unwanted feelings, others because "Mom always served these things together," and others because "my kids/partner only likes them this way."

✎📖 **Prompt: Create a list in your notebook called "My beliefs about food, eating and my weight."** Let your mind run free. This could be three separate lists or all jumbled into one.

- **Food:** What foods do you eat often and what ones do you avoid? Why? Do you have certain beliefs that lead you to make those choices?

- **Eating:** Do you have beliefs about what time or what sort of foods constitute breakfast? Or beliefs about when it's OK to have dessert or a bed-time snack? Beliefs (rules) about food waste or leaving food on your plate? Is it rude not to eat when others are eating?
- **Your weight:** Do you have beliefs like, "All the women in my family are fat"? Or about the impossibility of losing those last 20 pounds. Do you believe fat people are unlovable or undeserving?

Feel free to observe other people's behavior and see if you can discern what *their* beliefs might be. Once you begin seeing how many beliefs rule your food choices, eating behavior, and weight, you have to laugh at how varied, creative, and sneaky some of them are.

REMEMBER THIS

- Your beliefs are an invisible veil that clouds your perspective.
- Once you believe something to be true, you ignore evidence that disagrees.
- "Argue for your limitations, and sure enough, they're yours."

14

Standards: The Shoulds and the Shouldn'ts

Are you carrying around a head stuffed with *shoulds* and *shouldn'ts*? Tell me about it! I like to blame my perfectionist tendencies on my mother who was big on them (I want to say she was a *shoulder*, but the word reads as a body part). She had very high standards for her firstborn, from how I dressed or fixed my hair to my musical tastes and the friends I chose. As a parent myself, I now understand where she was coming from; she wanted me to succeed (and also not embarrass the family). However, my kid-self translated the message as, *You're not good enough*.

When I'd try to call her out on her criticisms she'd exclaim, "Don't be silly. You're perfect just as you are." Well, if I was so perfect, how come it seemed I never met her standards? For that matter, how come I always fell short on the standards I absorbed over the years from my peers, teachers, bosses, the general culture, the mass media? I didn't realize the extent to which these externally created standards were shaping how I felt about myself.

Standards. Says Who?

We think of a standard as something determined to be the norm by society. The way "they" say it should be. But who are "they"? Who gets to determine that their standards are the right ones for us? A standard is dependent on time, place, culture, and someone's judgments. For example, take what constitutes a beautiful woman. In the 1950s, curvaceous Marilyn Monroe and Sophia Loren were our beauties. In classical art, the beautiful woman was often downright plump, because plump meant healthy and nubile. Today, she's often an anorexic or photo-shopped model, although the pendulum seems to be swinging in the other direction, thanks to celebrities like Amy Schumer, Aidy Bryant, Lizzo, Mindy Kaling, Serena Williams and Sonya Renee Taylor.

Standards aren't all bad; we need them when it comes to objects that require common understanding, like how many ounces are in a quart or the particular formula for a chemical compound. In contrast, though, personal qualities are relative and always depend on comparison.

When we compare ourselves to others and judge ourselves harshly, we forget that those others may be putting forth their best selves to cover their own harsh self-judgments that we aren't privy to. Teddy Roosevelt once said, "Comparison is the thief of joy." That hit home with me, partly because Joy is my name, and also because comparisons never made me feel good. My negativity bias kept me focused on the many areas where I believed I fell short.

Comparison also made it painful when I was learning a new skill, because I would compare my current fumbling performance with what I thought it *should* be, once I mastered it. Shouldn't I get better faster, sooner, more consistently?

Shame

It's one thing to fall short of the standards we set for ourselves. It's quite another when we add shame to the mix. Even if you weren't raised as a Christian, the specter of "original sin" weighs heavily in American culture. Thanks to Adam and Eve, who *ate the forbidden fruit* (like chocolate and Cheetos today), some of us have come to believe we have a built-in urge to do bad things. The desires of the flesh—our appetites for sex and food—are evidence of our shameful nature. These desires should be tamped down or even eliminated. We must atone for our sins.

But has shaming yourself ever helped you lose weight? As Lindy West writes in her book, *Shrill,* "Shame contributes measurably to weight gain, not weight loss. Loving yourself is not antithetical to health, it is intrinsic to health. You can't take good care of a thing you hate."

Along the same vein, writer and teacher Geneen Roth says in her bestseller, *Women Food and God,* "For some reason, we are truly convinced that if we criticize ourselves, the criticism will lead to change. If we are harsh, we believe we will end up being kind. If we shame ourselves, we believe we end up loving ourselves. It has never been true, not for a moment, that shame leads to love. Only love leads to love."

✎📖 **Prompt: Have you shamed yourself?** Have you been made to feel guilty or ashamed because of your appetites or your size? Have other people called you names that made you feel bad about yourself? Have you called yourself shaming names? Make a list of these things on a separate sheet of paper. Write down all that garbage talk. All of it. Then review your list and notice if that shame ever changed your behavior for the better? *Now tear your list into little bits, or better yet, take a match to it and burn it!* (Outside, please.)

Your fat-mindset scolds, *You should have lost that weight by now.* I know. You tried hard. And some of the things you did (diets) worked for a bit. Then you stopped doing those things, and here you are, feeling defeated before you even get rolling. It's like you're dragging a donkey cart behind you, and you've piled every *perceived* failure from your past into it. With each perceived failure, the cart gets heavier and heavier. At some point your "logical" (if unconscious) conclusion is that failure is inevitable.

Since you're bound to fail, the best you can do is make half-assed gestures in the general direction of your goal. "At least I'm trying," you tell yourself. Well, *trying* won't even get you a cup of coffee—nor will *wishing* or *resolving* or *praying*. To get a cup of coffee, you need to reach into your wallet and pay the barista. Action.

All those times you missed the mark are in the past. Done. Gone. The past you remember (by which I mean the story you've told yourself about your past) doesn't predict the future. It doesn't mean you'll never get to your goal. It simply means that different actions are in order.

Radical thought: Perhaps you actually succeeded! Let's play *what if* with flipping the failure narrative. What if you *subconsciously intended* to create this weight problem and keep it around for a while? What if your weight problem was a convenient solution to an entirely different problem?

What? That's crazy talk! However, since you're the one who got yourself to where you are today, can you imagine the possibility that your weight issue has been useful to you in some way?

To explore this "*what if*_____," I invite you to do a short meditation I call, **"I did it myself!"** Please allow me to guide you rather than reading the transcript.

Guided Meditation: "I Did It Myself!" Set aside 15 minutes to do the meditation and note-taking. Images and experiences may pop immediately into mind. You also may draw some blanks or get unexpected, seemingly unrelated images and memories. It's all good. Take what you get.

Prompt: "I did it myself!" In your notebook, jot down what you noticed in this meditation. The two questions were, "What I did to create my weight problem." and "How my weight problem has been useful to me."

You're not bad, wrong, weak-willed, or a failure. Millions have found themselves in this same predicament. You did the best you could, given what you knew at the time. In each moment you chose to do what seemed least uncomfortable because that's what we humans do. That was then; this is now. As you become more aware of your fat machinery you gain more power over your ability to make fresh choices in the present moment.

• • • • • REMEMBER THIS • • • • •

- The standards you're trying to meet may not be your own.
- Shame is a toxic emotion. You're not a sinner; you're *human*.
- Just because you missed the mark in the past doesn't mean you'll never get there. It simply means that different actions are necessary.

15

Protection Scam

We all have tender spots in our psyches. Some of us harbor much worse than tender—truly horrible things have happened to us. We don't want to feel that pain again, so we do whatever we can to avoid poking that particular bear. Instead, we become the unwitting prisoner of our remembered past. However, as Anais Nin wrote, "And the day came when the risk to remain tight in a bud was more painful than the risk it took to blossom." I believe this with all my heart.

When you completed the meditation and prompt, **"I did it myself!"** in the previous chapter, you considered how your weight problem might have solved a different problem. It could be serving subconsciously to protect you from a re-exposure to old pain. The "awful thing" may have happened when you were relatively slim, so maintaining a blanket of blubber could be a strategy to prevent a recurrence of the awful thing. For others, the obsession with eating and dieting serves a different purpose—to leave no room for experiencing negative emotions such as grief, fear, guilt, and shame.

In my case, those emotions coalesced around what I convinced myself was my unacceptable behavior during the last year of my husband's life. I had been an impatient, grudging nurse and an unresponsive lover who was turned off by his emaciated appearance at a time he most needed physical affection. Then, after Edward died, I acted as if all was going just fine, dutifully putting on a chirpy cheerful, business-as-usual show for the sake of the kids. I stuffed my grief at his death, I stuffed my shame at falling short as a wife, and I stuffed my terror of facing the future as a single mother with no discernible job skills.

As long as I could be preoccupied 24/7 with losing weight and all it entailed—planning the next diet, figuring out how to cheat on it, and the subsequent self-hatred when I did cheat or quit—there was no space to confront my unacceptable emotions.

It was a perfect protection scam, until it wasn't. I call it a *scam*, because our cover-up behaviors never really work, do they? The truth wants out, and it always finds a way.

Facts or Interpretation?

Here's the crazy thing. The truth is rarely the story we've been telling ourselves. Certain specific things happened, which a video camera could record—these are the *facts*. Then we began to spin our *interpretations*, adding cause, blame, and emotion. According to neurological research, the pain of the moment is extremely short-lived; what lingers in the mind are our interpretations—our technicolor stories and feelings about what happened. As time passes, the story gets further edited. Certain details are minimized or discarded and other elements are magnified to solidify our preferred narrative. Take my "fat story" from Camp Wyonegonic, which placed the blame for my weight gain on my Mom-caused misery, until my recent discovery of the camp director's report to my parents, revealing that quite possibly I'd spun a convenient fiction.

The facts of my situation in 1975 were this: My husband, Edward, got cancer, went through many unpleasant treatments while continuing to run his business, and after two difficult years, he died. At the same time, I had two preschoolers to care for, plus a home and garden to oversee. Edward and I were both stressed by the situation, as neither of us had ever dealt with terminal illness or raising two small kids.

These facts happened and were unchangeable. The story I kept retelling myself (my *interpretation*) was that I was a terrible wife, a poor mother, and an all-around bad person. That story kept me stuck. I used it to avoid feeling sad at our immense loss and to avoid taking the scary steps required to create a new life. Obsessing about my weight took so much of my energy that it "solved" that problem.

When I faced the reality of my situation, I saw that I had a choice in how to conduct my life going forward. The "obstacle" (that crazy-making weight I'd gained) revealed itself as the path toward resolving not only my own weight problems, but also helping others who were caught in the same demoralizing loop.

The following prompt is a further exploration of "**I did it myself!**"

✎📖 **Prompt: Do you have a protection scam?** Are you maintaining a blubber blanket to protect yourself from imagined harm? Or are you the weight-obsessive type who uses food to stuff unwanted feelings? You certainly could be both. In your notebook, blurt your thoughts onto the page without thought or judgment. Before you begin to answer these questions, close your eyes and allow yourself a minute to go back in time to revisit this moment (or moments).

- Did something bad or painful happen in your thinner past that you do not want repeated? What were *the facts* of that situation? (Facts = what a video camera would observe, not your dramatization and interpretations.) List the facts: this happened, then this happened, then this…
- Did you make a decision at that time in order to prevent a recurrence—that from then on, you'd always (or never) behave a certain way or be a particular kind of person? If you eat or worry about your weight instead of feeling negative emotions, do you know what feelings you're avoiding? Be specific: what, when, where?
- How is your protection scam working? How is it failing you?
- What do you believe might happen if you allowed yourself to feel some of these stuffed feelings?

Once you notice and articulate these old stories, you can reexamine them.

- In reconsidering this event, can you distinguish between the facts and your emotional interpretations?
- If you were a kid when the event happened, is it possible your interpretation was based on a child's very limited perspective? If it happened today, would you interpret it differently?
- If you were to look at the event *from the other person's point of view* and imagine what was going on *for them*, might you see it differently now?
- With the benefit of hindsight, did you do the best you could at the time?
- Knowing what you know now, could you forgive yourself? (If not, what would it take?)

It's a Racket

The additional fallout from maintaining a protection scam is that it gets you off the hook from owning up to your responsibility in maintaining a problem. You can blame outside forces for your troubles. You've got a good story, and you're sticking to it! But it's a racket, with short-term benefits and long-term costs.

Why would anyone hold on to a racket that maintains the very problem you claim you want to resolve? Ha! The $64,000 question. It's all about the *payoff*, the "benefit" you get from running the racket. The payoff is that you get to be right or make others wrong. For example, if your racket is *the last ten pounds are impossible to lose*, you get to be right if you quit the diet at ten pounds from goal. Or let's say you baked brownies "for the kids," then ate half of them; you can blame the kids for your weakness. If your racket is *no one loves a fat person*, are you the one keeping people at arms' length?

Can you see how this works? Your racket becomes a self-fulfilling prophecy and keeps you stuck. You can feel righteous about the persistence of your problem, but the cost—your results, your self-esteem, your autonomy, your freedom, your happiness—is steep. As Henry David Thoreau once said, "The cost of a thing is the amount of what I will call life which is required to be exchanged for it, immediately or in the long run."

No one says you have to drop your racket. Feel free to hang on to it as long as you wish. But now that you recognize you may be running a racket, you're no longer in a rut with no options. You're back in the driver's seat with the ability to choose: continue as before, or explore a different path. That choice is up to you.

REMEMBER THIS

- Your cover-up behaviors never really work. Bite the bullet and look deep.
- The truth (the facts) is rarely the story you've been telling yourself.
- Once you recognize the payoff you get from your protection scam, the jig is up.

16

Body Break I: '*Preshurate* Your Body

To lose confidence in one's body is to lose confidence in oneself.
—Simone de Beauvoir

I'm sure you treat the people you respect with care and concern for their well-being. Do you treat *your body* in that kindly way? It's time to become more attentive to this essential relationship.

These two body appreciation practices are quick and simple. Neither takes more than five minutes. Once you get the hang of them, feel free to improvise. If you can make each one a daily practice, you'll feel a closer connection to your body. I promise your body will be grateful too.

Practice: Waking up *with* your body. This simple practice will start your day on a positive note and create a more appreciative relationship with the vehicle that gives you life. Set your alarm for five minutes earlier than usual and spend those minutes, still cozy under the covers, greeting your body. "Hi, body," you might say. "We're in this thing for the long haul; thanks for joining me here today."

Start at your toes. Wiggle them, saying. "Hi, toes." Rotate your ankles: "Good morning, ankles." So far so good—you can do this! Shift your knees to one side, then the other: "Hello, sweet knees." Gradually move segment by segment up to your head, wiggling and greeting every part. Now stretch as far as you can on each side, making a C-shape of your body. Put your hands on your heart and thank it for continuing to beat without your having to ask. Take several slow deep breaths and thank your loyal lungs. Enjoy a loud, luxurious yawn. Finally, give your scalp a quick massage (like a mock shampoo) to wake up the hardworking brain within.

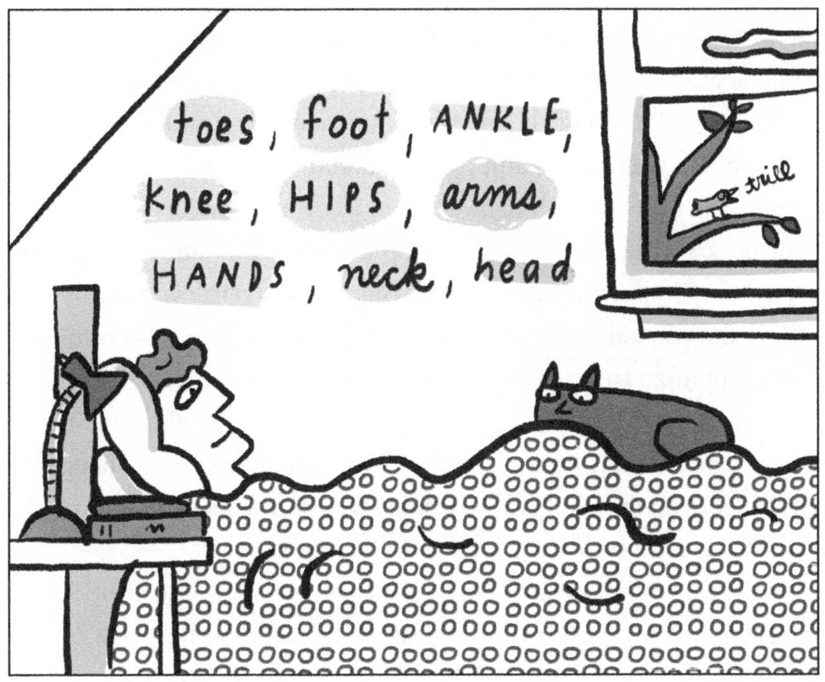

Practice: Ending the day with gratitude. There's a delicious moment at the end of the day when you slither beneath the sheets and let your body sink into the mattress. *Ahhhh.* You're totally supported and weightless at the same time. Nothing more to do. Let that shit go.

Well, one more thing—*'preshurate* your body. (That's how my toddler son used to pronounce *appreciate*, and our family still pronounces it that way.)

Your body has carried you around for hours, enabling you to work, think, love, feel, and be. At the very least, it deserves a couple of minutes of your *'preshuration*, and gratitude.

So, stretch out, face up on the bed. Allow each part of your body to sink deeply into the mattress, especially your head and neck. Turn your head from side to side, then open and shut your jaw a few times to make sure your neck is as loose as possible.

Take five slow breaths and feel yourself just *being*. Repeat the same toe-to-head routine you did in the morning, adding an expression of genuine gratitude for each part. Be generous with your praise. I mean, think about it! The body is a miracle in so many dimensions. It conveys you from here to there (thank you, legs and feet), it manipulates objects (thank you, arms and hands), your butt lets you sit on its cushion, and your neck spends the day holding up a heavy head jam-packed with thoughts—Command Central for all that's going on below. Your mouth tastes, your nose smells, your ears hear, and your brain sorts a continuous barrage of input to make sense of it all. Wow!

Don't forget your trunk, which houses so many crucial organs: heart, lungs, digestive tract, reproductive organs. Holy crap, it's mind boggling, all that goes on in there. Where would the food you love to eat go if you had no digestive system? Some gratitude, please.

How fortunate you are to exist! Give yourself a big hug of *'preshuration*, then give your body the gift of sleep. Repeat nightly.

• • • • • REMEMBER THIS • • • • •

- Your body has been either ignored or unloved too long.
- Talk to your body as you'd talk to someone you love.
- And mean it.

17

Rate Your Food: SuperTool #4

Most of our assumptions have
outlived their uselessness.
—Marshall McLuhan

To release excess pounds, I knew that I'd to have to eat less. But how could I do this without feeling deprived, the way I always did when I was on a diet? My daughter, Heather, who was seven at the time, gave me the answer. Become a picky eater. Don't waste precious calories on inferior food.

In fairness, Heather wasn't a *picky* eater; she was a *discriminating* eater. She wasn't blinded by prior assumptions about how a food should taste. She judged the food in her mouth on its own merits.

Here's how the idea for SuperTool #4 came to me:

My Carrot Epiphany

For an afternoon snack, I'd set out a small plate of carrot sticks. Heather took a bite of one stick and refused to eat any more of them.

"Hey," I said. "You like carrots. They're sweet and crunchy."

"Not this one," she said, pushing her plate toward me. "It's dry. And it isn't sweet either."

I reached across the counter to try one for myself. She was right. It sat like tasteless cardboard in my mouth (not that I'd ever eaten cardboard, but I could imagine it). Hmph! What do you know—a carrot that did not live up to my expectations.

This troubled me. How did I think a carrot would taste? Did I even notice when it didn't taste or feel as I expected? And if it wasn't up to snuff, did I eat it anyway? Of course I did. It was a carrot! I had a belief formed decades ago that carrots were sweet, crunchy, and good for me. After that, I must have stopped experiencing them, instead eating memories of that original carrot, which might have been from Daddy's garden.

Oops. This was a different vegetable. I spit it out. If I were to rate it on a scale of 1 to 10—1 being yuck! And 10 being YUM!—this carrot rated a 2 at best.

I pulled several more carrots from the fridge for a taste test. I peeled one from the bunch I'd served Heather and one from a fresher bunch. I enlisted my senses of sight, smell, and touch as well as taste. The carrot from the tired bunch didn't have the wet sheen under the peel like the newer one did. It arched slightly, whereas the newer one broke when I tried bending it. The newer one smelled earthy and carroty; as I chomped down on it, its sweetness spread quickly to my tongue. Heather's had no odor, juice, sweetness, or flavor. No wonder she didn't want it.

For someone who claimed to love food, I had deluded myself. I wasn't tasting the food in my mouth; I was *tasting my belief* about it, based on some earlier experience. Long ago, I decided carrots "tasted good" and were "good for you," regardless of the evidence in my mouth.

Just as each person is unique, so is each humble carrot. And every other food.

A Chocolate Disappointment

What about sweet treats I loved, like chocolate? I love anything and everything chocolate—or so I told myself. I had called myself a "chocoholic" for years, rarely stopping to discern whether it was any good. To test myself, I found some Hershey's Kisses left over from Easter. Normally, I'd free the candy from the foil and pop it into my mouth. In a couple of chews it would be gone, and I'd be ready for another. This time, I took my time and focused on every sensory aspect of the Kiss.

First, I noticed that the mere sight of the shiny wrap caused my salivary glands to spurt. It set my heart beating a bit faster. I slowly pulled its paper tab and, like a strip tease, peeled back the foil a little at a time, gradually revealing the waxy brown mountain inside. I stroked it with my index finger to see if it felt as waxy as it looked. It did. Not so appealing. I smelled it. Huh. It even smelled a bit waxy, with just a hint of cocoa. I licked it. It took several seconds for the exterior to melt enough that any flavor reached my tongue.

I was surprised that the first flavor I registered was a slight sourness, followed by a cloying sweetness. It wasn't until I bit off a third of the Kiss and pressed it into the roof of my mouth that I tasted any chocolate flavor at all. I let the bite melt and slowly trickle down my throat. At this point I rated it about halfway between yuck and yum.

After I swallowed, I waited for any lingering flavor. What lingered was sourness, a sourness that made me want to cover it by taking another bite. Instead I marched over to my trusty garbage can and tossed it in. My rating plummeted.

How many precious calories had I wasted on mediocre chocolate? No more!

Next, I decided to taste test some brownies. I made a batch from scratch, using the recipe on the back of the can of cocoa, and compared it to a batch I made from a mix. The difference in texture (crumby versus chewy) and flavor intensity was dramatic. Having done that test, I can now tell at first bite if a brownie is for real. I have not eaten a brownie from a box mix since.

Very recently I learned why my expectations and taste buds didn't align. My brain had already made up its mind and left the building. Fascinating new research in neuroscience has discovered that the brain is not so much *reactive* to all the sensory data coming in as it is *predictive*. Guessing what might happen next on the basis of prior similar experiences is a more efficient use of its energy budget. In my case (eating carrots or chocolate), my brain expects that the experience will be pleasurable, so it doesn't pay much attention to the reality in my mouth unless it's markedly different—or I'm really focused on the experience.

The fact that the same food could rate differently at different stages of consumption was my other big aha! For example, in first looking at the Hershey's Kiss, I had high expectations of how it would taste. If it were on a scale of 1 to 10, I expected an 8 or 9. But my first bite rated about a 3 because I had trouble getting past the waxiness. Middle bite when the chocolate flavor became more apparent? 6. Last bite? 8. Mouth taste about a minute after I finished? Sour -1. I also discovered that even something as yummy as the brownie-from-scratch, which started at 10, dropped down to 6 at the last bite—not because the flavor had changed, but because my taste buds got bored.

Furthermore, the same food could rate differently depending on how hungry I was. For example, trail mix isn't very interesting, but after I'd just hiked five miles up a mountain, every raisin or peanut tasted amazing.

Food Rating—SuperTool #4

Since I wanted to become a more discriminating eater, rating my food seemed like the best way to begin. It gave me something useful to focus on as I ate, woke up my taste buds, and as a pleasing byproduct, it made me a better cook.

Do not skip this exercise.

✏📖 **Prompt: Rate your food.** For the next week, keep a simple food diary that just lists each food as you eat it and your rating of it, using a scale of 1 to 10, 1 being Yuck! and 10 being Yum! (Anything from 1 to 4 is probably not worth the caloric input, and you might consider setting it aside.) If you want to make the exercise more interesting, you could enter three numbers: a rating for how you expect the food to taste before you bite it, one for the first bite, and one for the last bite.

Rate Your Food Chart

Rate from 1-10, 1=yuck, 5=passable, 10=fantastic

	Expectation	First bite	Last bite
Brownie from scratch	10	10	6
Kale Salad	5	4	7
Black bean chilli	6	7	4

Taste Tests Bring Your Senses into the Present Moment

Repeat the following taste test frequently over the next few months, substituting different types of foods—some you eat often, some that you consider special treats, some that relate to childhood memories, comfort foods, favorite snacks. Then you can expand the test to foods you've never eaten before (new vegetables, foreign dishes, and the like). Set aside time for these taste tests when you won't be distracted. One or two items to taste test per day is fine. (In these taste tests, we always call food "the item" to detach our minds from any prior associations with "carrot," "fudge," "mac and cheese," etc.) You're going to approach the item as if you had dropped in from Mars and never been exposed to it before.

Practice: Mindful taste tests. Choose from a few foods you eat often enough that you probably no longer taste them in the present moment—carrot sticks, celery, slices from different types of apples, saltines, potato chips, pickles, slices of cheese, whatever you have on hand. Here's how to proceed:

1. Before taking a bite, explore the item with all your other senses: examine it from all sides, sniff it, feel it. Does it remind you of anything? Does it bring up memories? Do you have an expectation about how it will taste?

2. Record your thoughts in your notebook.
3. Lick the item. Do you get any flavor? Describe it.
4. Take a bite of the item, but do not chew yet. How does it feel in your mouth? Move it to different places in your mouth to see if flavor is based on location. Do you taste any flavor yet? In what part of your mouth? Do you get a sense of freshness or staleness?
5. Chomp once with your molars. Is the flavor stronger or different? What is the predominant flavor? Is it sweet, salty, sour, bitter, savory? What is the texture? Do you like it? Does it make a pleasing noise in your head?
6. Now chew without swallowing (as best you can) until all the flavor seems extracted.
7. Swallow (or spit the food into a napkin) and let your mouth remain empty for at least fifteen seconds. Is there an aftertaste? Some foods have an imperceptibly unpleasant aftertaste that makes you want another bite to refresh the mouth (those Kisses). Spicy foods also prompt the mouth to want more.
8. Record your additional observations in your notebook.

Most of us eat from a surprisingly limited repertoire of foods, which we've eaten hundreds or thousands of times over the years. Our preferences, opinions, and beliefs about food come from way back in time. Once I set aside my assumptions and expectations, I opened my mind up to trying foods that I'd decided years earlier I didn't like—olives, eggplant, peppers, squash, parsley, coconut, licorice. I still detest licorice, but everything else tasted suprisingly good.

Additional taste test explorations

Seasonal variation. Foods vary widely depending on the season and how well or long they've been stored, so taste test the same food in different seasons. Cruciferous vegetables like broccoli and kale, for example, are sweeter in the colder months. A strawberry or tomato in season is nothing like its tasteless winter version.

Comparative tests. Pretend you're on a taste-testing panel at *Cooks Illustrated,* comparing different versions of the same food. Try several kinds of apple, several types of cracker, vinegars, olive oils, brown versus white rice and long-grain versus short grain. Try chocolate bars with different percentages of cocoa, milk versus dark, expensive versus cheap, packaged cake or brownie mixes versus those made from scratch.

Name the ingredients. When you eat an interesting food at a friend's house or a restaurant—something that you didn't prepare—slow way down and try to figure out what the ingredients are. Is it pork or chicken? Is that garlic or onion? Sugar or honey? Is it made with butter or olive oil? What spices or herbs are in it? What else does it remind you of? Could you duplicate it in your kitchen, and if so, how might you alter it? I made this a detective game for my kids; it was a sneaky way to introduce new foods and train their taste buds. It paid off; today they're all fantastic cooks (and slim, too).

• • • • • REMEMBER THIS • • • • •

- Familiarity breeds unconsciousness.
- Training your taste buds takes regular practice.
- Mindful eating is more pleasurable eating.

PART FOUR

Awaken Your Goal-Mindset

In this important section, you'll understand why the freedom you seek requires you to shift your self-image. You'll experience a healthy aspect of your identity that has been dormant for too long, thanks to your negativity bias. (Your fat-mindset will resist this shift. Fear not, we'll address resistance in Part Five.)

The concepts of "growth mindset" and "fixed mindset" were popularized in the 2007 book, *Mindset: The New Psychology of Success*, by Stanford professor, Carol Dweck. Her studies indicated that how you view your identity shapes how you behave, which shapes the direction of your future. If you believe in your ability to change and grow, it creates a sense of possibility and motivates you to keep going, regardless of setbacks.

18

A Question of Identity

Life isn't about finding yourself. Life is about creating yourself.
—George Bernard Shaw

I bet you're sick of all this poking and prodding at your fat-mindset (machinery). As you're beginning to discern for yourself, assumptions and beliefs color our perception of reality. They're so much a part of how we think that we don't notice how much attention we give to the negative and how little attention we give to affirming our best selves.

Assumptions and beliefs help us make sense of the moment, and they give us a sense of order and predictability. At the same time, because they are based in the past and filter our vision, they constrict our ideas of what's possible.

At the core of these filters is *identity—who you think you are.*

Who Do You Think You Are?

Who you think you are shapes the direction of your life—your interests, lifestyle, career, hobbies, relationships, and so forth. Our identities are constructed not just from our innate capabilities and limitations, but from the stories we tell ourselves about who we are, as well as from the stories laid on us by our most influential mentors: parents, teachers, peers, and from cultural norms. In ways great and small, these stories determine the choices we believe are open (or closed) to us, and in turn influence the actions we take.

Growing up in a musical family made it easy for me to think of myself as a musician too, because it came easily to me, and my musician mother reinforced that story. At the same time, I convinced myself I was not artistic because I couldn't draw horses like my best friend, Barbara, and my fourth-grade teacher didn't hang my masterpiece in the school art show. As it all turned out, I quit nurturing my musician self (by not practicing—works every time!) and began nurturing my artistic self (taking classes, practicing) so those early identities have reversed themselves. Repeated actions create habits, and those habits lead us to believe we are a certain sort of person.

We each harbor many identities, some more dominant and developed than others, depending on the attention you give them. Math whiz, number numbskull, athlete, klutz, peacemaker, old fart, funny person, problem-solver, flaky, neat freak, disorganized, good parent, fat person, techie, teacher, psychic, loser, smart, dancer, shy, writer, boring, generous—the list of the stories we tell ourselves about our strengths and weaknesses is endless, and we play them out in our daily lives where they get reinforced by repetition. However—and most importantly—we also harbor identities as yet undiscovered.

✎📖 **Prompt: Who do you think you are? Who do you think you are *not*?** Make a list of all your identities—words you'd use to describe yourself. Then make a second list: who you think you are not. How have these identities been reinforced? How have some withered for lack of attention or conflicting evidence? Have any of your identities changed over time?

You picked up this book because one of your identities is "person with a weight problem." This is your fat-mindset talking. You've related to food, your body, and to dieting through the lens of someone who doesn't like their body size. Telling yourself this story has only made you feel bad about yourself, and it makes it hard to shake this entrenched identity.

But there is another possibility.

Life Is Not Either/Or

Some view the world in polar opposites—dualistic, either/or choices: good or bad, light or dark, hot or cold, masculine or feminine, fat or thin. However, you cannot have one without the other. Good only exists relative to bad. We cannot know hot unless we know cold, light without dark. Furthermore, none of these are true opposites; they're always on a continuum.

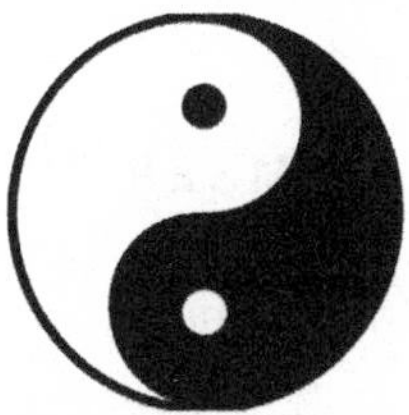

The Taoist yin-yang symbol represents this in graphic terms. Half is black and half is white, each containing the seed of the other. The halves are intertwined within a circle, as if each is growing into or becoming the other.

Consider this: within your fat-mindset lies the seed of your goal-mindset. It's impossible to hold this negative self-concept without also harboring its opposite. Like the yin-yang symbol, one calls forth the other. Unfortunately, you've given your fat-mindset an excess of attention.

Your brain is plastic, which means it is continually building new neural pathways and reinforcing older ones. The more frequently you repeat certain behaviors and thought patterns, the stronger the neural pathways become and the less energy the brain has to expend on the task. If you practice driving a car enough, the brain can relax and allow you to simultaneously talk to the person in the passenger seat or navigate the interchange. It's really quite remarkable.

Here's the bad news: when you "practice" your negative thoughts and counterproductive habits, you're automating and strengthening a neural rut in your brain, ready to encourage your worst eating impulses and to shame you for doing so.

The good news is the brain is still plastic. As you practice new thought and behavior patterns, the brain can and will build more supportive neural pathways to help you maintain a more positive self-image. The key, of course, is regular practice of these new skills and ways of thinking.

In the next chapter, we'll dissect the circular mechanism that creates a self-fulfilling prophecy out of the person you think you are—your created identity.

• • • • • REMEMBER THIS • • • • •

- Who you think you are shapes the direction of your life.
- Who you think you are *not* also shapes the direction of your life.
- Within your fat-mindset lies the seed of your goal-mindset.

19

The Cycle of Self-Fulfilling Prophecies

Decades ago, Werner Erhard introduced me to the **"Be ➤ Do ➤ Have"** model, which depicted the natural flow of creation—a resistance-free process for achieving a goal. It went something like this:

BE: Your identity, who you believe you are *or could be.* Which leads to…

DO: Actions, behaviors. Which lead to…

HAVE: Results, outcome.

For example:

- **BE/Identity/Belief.** Before I even started cooking, I believed I would be a good cook. I'd seen my mom create tasty meals with what *seemed* like little effort, so I could envision myself being a good cook too.
- **DO/Actions/Behaviors.** Believing that I would be a good cook, I took action. I acquired the gear I'd need to produce tasty meals—some pots, knives, and a couple of cookbooks. I tried new recipes with a spirit of curiosity and adventure. If the soufflé refused to rise, I laughed and just called it a frittata, then I figured out why it fell and fixed it next time. I kept practicing and learning.
- **HAVE/Results/Outcome.** I got the outcome I'd envisioned—strong skills and a reputation as a good cook. I mastered not only the

cheese soufflé but many other tricky dishes as well. I even worked for a couple of years as a food writer.

However, this model depicts a straight line, when in reality the process is circular, because the *results (HAVE)* come back around and reinforce who you think you are—your *identity (BE)*. Your identity becomes a self-fulfilling prophecy— a version of *confirmation bias*, which is the tendency to favor information that confirms our existing beliefs.

If I believe I'm a good cook, I dismiss my fallen soufflé as an expected part of the learning process. If instead I believed that cooking was too complicated for a klutz like me, my fallen soufflé would only prove my incompetence, and I would cease trying (in the unlikely event I attempted the soufflé in the first place). The cycle would turn in a negative direction.

[Word Choice Alert: I'm going to use the word "fat" here, because that's how our internal trash-talker talks. The internal trash-talker does not understand body positivity.]

Now let's see what happens when we plug into the cycle the belief, "I am fat:"

- **BE/Identity/Belief:** I am fat.
- **DO/Actions/Behaviors:** I go on a diet. I quit eating carbohydrates or follow another diet du jour.
- **HAVE/Results/Outcome:** However, because *in my mind* I have the belief "I am fat" (and because strict regimes are hard to sustain), sooner or later I fall off the diet and once again I have the extra pounds. So back around to…
- **BE/Identity/Belief:** ***I am fat.*** I've reinforced this negative belief, and the vicious cycle begins again.

I struggled with this kind of thinking ever since I gained those 25 pounds at camp as a teen. Dieters know it as the *yo-yo syndrome*, a common consequence of fat-mindset. This is one reason why people with anorexia never feel thin enough.

The Future as an Extension of our Past Experience

The human imagination is too often constrained by our limited view of what's possible. We default to an assumption that the future will unfold as an extension of what we've experienced so far. Sure, we'll get older, and we may get richer or poorer, healthier or sicker, slightly more or less successful—nevertheless *we expect the future to continue on a trajectory we can imagine*. We have no contingency plan for lightning strikes or alien abduction, because they seem implausible.

My own blinkered vision of the future—my Perfect Life Plan as envisioned by me at 18—was an updated extension of how I saw my mother's life. Meet Prince Charming, get married, become skilled in the housewifely arts (give me a break; I was born in 1940), have two perfect children and maybe a creative side hustle, live happily ever after. When Edward got sick and died at 31, the rupture in my reality forced me to rethink *everything*.

Absent such a rupture to shake you awake, you must recognize that you've been projecting your future out of what you've experienced in the past. To create a fresh future—in this case, a future in which you're free of weight worries—the first step is to become aware that you've been projecting your never-slim future out of your old weight war stories.

To make this shift, you have *to imagine the possibility that there's another way* to create the future you'd prefer—life as a person who is at peace with food and their body, and at a body size they feel good about. Your identity undergoes a complete paradigm pivot. Once you experience this, you have the freedom and power to create a more helpful narrative in each present moment—and a future no longer dictated by the past.

- **BE/Identity/Belief:** I am at my right weight and am at peace with food and my body. [*Your own words…*]
- **DO/Actions/Behaviors:** I only eat when I'm hungry, and I stop well before I'm full. I slowly savor my food. I eat what I like and toss what I don't want.
- **HAVE/Results/Outcome:** A trimmer body, a goal-mindset, freedom from weight worries, moving on to other projects, *(Your own words)*. And back around to…
- **BE/Identity/Belief:** I am at my right weight and am at peace with food and my body.

With each little success, you reinforce your positive identity. New neural pathways begin to strengthen in your brain.

"Sure, right, fine," I hear you thinking. "Easy for you to say, but I can't just press a magic button and presto-change-o think of myself as being at my ideal weight and free of weight worries."

Stay tuned. In the next two chapters we will pull that rabbit out of the hat.

• • • • • REMEMBER THIS • • • • •

- The future rarely unfolds in a straight line.
- Your future is created by your beliefs about who you are and what you're capable of.
- Your current actions are the key to the future you.

20

What Is Goal-Mindset?

The real voyage of discovery consists not in seeking new landscapes but in having new eyes.
—Marcel Proust

My breakfast with Carol lacked the observable drama of an earthquake, yet in my head tectonic plates shifted. As I observed her nonchalant attitude toward her piece of cherry pie, I realized not everyone related to food the way I did. I decided the only way to understand these people I called "true thins" back in the 1970s was to observe them at meals, at parties, and with their kids. I also grilled them about their food preferences and attitudes. Today I call this constellation of "true thin" attitudes and eating behaviors "goal-mindset."

I began to see some common threads among "true thins:"

- If they weren't hungry, they had no problem ignoring edible offerings.
- As soon as they felt satisfied, they stopped eating, even if it meant tossing good food in the garbage.
- They were patient enough to wait for the entire meal to be laid out attractively before diving in.
- They paid little attention to caloric or carbohydrate counts unless they had a medical condition like diabetes or heart disease.
- They ate foods they liked and ignored foods they didn't like—no

guilt and no obligation to please the cook or maintain membership in the Clean Plate Club.

- They rarely thought about food between meals.
- They were unconcerned about appropriateness. Pizza for breakfast, Cheerios for supper? Sure.
- They didn't seem emotionally invested in what they were eating. It wasn't a substitute for love, excitement, comfort, or Mom; it was just food.
- When they were bored, stressed, angry, procrastinating, sad, lonely, etc. they did not run to food.

How true thins stuffed those ubiquitous human feelings? I had no idea. Chew their fingernails to a nub? Smoke? Dig dandelions? Bite the heads off kittens? I never got around to doing this part of the research.

Although their attitudes and behaviors at first seemed alien to me, I realized most babies, including my own, ate like true thins. They liked what they liked and didn't like what they didn't like. When they didn't like something or weren't hugry—pffft! They spit it out and clamped their little lips together so no more could get in. I realized I'd had occasional moments of acting like a thin person too—when I was engrossed or upset or disliked the food being offered.

Becoming someone who no longer thinks of themselves as "having a weight problem" is not as remote a reach as you've feared. Behavioral economist Katy Milkman, author of the bestseller, *How to Change: The Science of Getting from Where You Are to Where You Want to Be,* reports great success with the technique she calls "copy and paste." In other words, find someone who has mastered the skill or behavior you're working on, and imitate their methods. That's what I was doing when I asked myself, "WWCD?" (What would Carol do?) And that's what this important meditation and prompt is all about.

Guided Meditation: Your "True Thin" Friends. Set aside at least 15 minutes to do this meditation and write up your observations. As you bring these people to mind, you may wonder if the person actually suffers from fat-mindset and is just putting on a good show. It doesn't matter. Just take the images you get.

Prompt: Goal-mindset ("true thin") behaviors and attitudes. On a fresh page in your notebook, start a list titled "Goal-Mindset Behaviors and Attitudes." Write down specifics you noticed in the meditation. Then go back to what you wrote about your friends with weight issues (chapter 12) and see if some of their behaviors could be listed in opposite form. (Example: "If it's edible, they eat everything on their plate," becomes "They're picky and only eat what they like.")

REMEMBER THIS

- Become a careful observer of how, what, and when other people eat.
- Learn from those who already have it together.
- Imitation is the sincerest form of flattery.

21

The Wall Comes Down

The whole life of the individual is nothing but the process of giving birth to oneself.
—Erich Fromm

BEing "fat" is an acquired belief, a story you've told yourself and acted out for a long time. Through repetition, your brain has laid down connections, making it your default mode.

The shift to being content with your weight is not about what you weigh (though you will drop pounds if that's part of your goal). It's about how you think of yourself and how that self-image reinforces itself in your behaviors in ways big and small every day.

For example, let's give each of two women a piece of chocolate cake. *Both women are at their ideal weight, but one thinks of herself as slim and the other thinks of herself as fat.* For Ms. Slim-Mind, the cake is a delight to be savored. For Ms. Fat-Mind, the cake is a sin; it must be wolfed down before anyone notices, especially herself.

The experience of eating the cake is different in two important ways: 1) the story the eater tells themselves about it and 2) the pleasure each allows themselves.

It may seem like a giant leap of faith to imagine you could change your identity from fat-mindset to goal-mindset. However, just as your malleable brain created the rut of fat-thinking that's kept you stuck, it can and will create new neural connections to strengthen your new self-image. With mindful practice of the tools in this book, the transformation is absolutely within your power.

Remember the story of the Cherokee chief who had two metaphorical wolves inside? You are now ready to meet your inner "wolf" and free this self from the shackles of your fat-mindset past so you can begin to nurture your liberated self with fresh ideas.

DO NOT SKIP THE FOLLOWING MEDITATION. It will help you get more in touch with your goal-mind self and with the barriers you've put between yourself and that self. It is an essential turning point as you transform your mindset. ***Please listen rather than read, so your imagination is free to roam.***

Guided Meditation: The Wall Comes Down. Give yourself a half-hour when you will not be disturbed. You may experience a variety of emotions during the process, like sadness or anger or amusement. Whatever comes up, just allow it to be there. And whatever you see or create during the process is perfect; there is no correct vision, no correct way to do this. Pantomiming your creation with hand gestures helps make it real.

Prompt: The Mending Wall. Take several minutes to write in your notebook all the jumbled thoughts that came up during the meditation. You may not have emerged from behind the wall as the radiant slim king or queen of your dreams, but you have now had the experience that you were the one who created that wall, and that you have the power to demolish it. Then, take another few minutes to respond to these famous lines from Robert Frost's famous poem "The Mending Wall":

> *Before I built a wall I'd ask to know*
> *What I was walling in, or walling out,*
> *And to whom I was like to give offense.*
> *Something there is that doesn't love a wall,*
> *That wants it down.*

• • • • • REMEMBER THIS • • • • •

- Your wall is a constructed thing.
- You built your wall because you believed it kept you "safe."
- You can tear down your wall and step into your future.

22

From Discipline to Devotion

It does not matter how slowly you go,
as long as you do not stop.
—Confucius

Let's review what we've covered so far. My intention has been to guide you through some pretty major mental shifts in reframing how you view yourself, your weight, and your locus of control (who's boss). Some of these shifts are well underway, and we're just launching others:

- From problem to project
- From spectator to participant
- From judge to curious observer
- From diet rigidity to mindful choosing
- From food as danger to food as nourishing pleasure
- From fat-mindset to goal-mindset
- From negative self-talk to affirming the positive

By now, you've probably begun to recognize some of your less-than-helpful strategies for dealing with your weight "problem." You've learned how to use some of the most critical tools in this book's arsenal—you've tuned up your internal fuel gauge, you've awakened your palate by rating your food, and you're using the Winning Formula from chapter 11 every day to become more present to your food. (You *are* using the Winning Formula, aren't you? If not, why not?)

You've also begun to shift how you *perceive* your weight issue by observing your fat-mindset and its stories, and you've met your inner ideal-sized self. These shifts lead to more effective *actions.* You're making great progress, and I applaud you!

Now I want to add one more shift... from thinking of this process as a ***discipline***—enforced compliance, which triggers resistance—to ***a way of expressing devotion***—to your body, to your health, to the food that gives you life, to your sanity and your future. As you read or reread each chapter, consider recasting each exercise as a form of devotional as well.

Like learning any new skill, mastery only comes with daily practice over the long haul. Even when you reach whatever you named as your goal, the devotional practice continues. A true practice has no endpoint; we do it every day because it feels good and because it works.

• • • • • REMEMBER THIS • • • • •

- This mindfulness process is a way of expressing devotion to your body, your food, your health, your sanity, and your future.
- Shift your attitude ➤ shift your actions ➤ shift your life.

23

You Deserve a Pretty Plate

We eat first with our eyes.
—Apicius, First century Roman

We sometimes forget that *all* of our senses are involved in the enjoyment of a meal, not just taste and smell. For example, imagine eating a potato chip that's gone soggy—you still have the salt, fat, and flavor, but without that crunchy sound and the sensation of shattering between your teeth, the chip is inedible.

Do you remember school cafeteria food? The grayish brown heap we called mystery meat! The appearance of food on your plate affects your pleasure more than you might think.

I observed this for the first time on an April Fools' Day when I was about ten. My mother (aka "the Human Garbage Pail") swore that she could eat any food, as long as it was not spoiled. My sisters and I decided to put her claim to the test. We shut her out of the kitchen while we (with Daddy's help) prepared a special meal for her, giggling with the audacity of our plan.

Our menu consisted of foods that were white to begin with. To each we added a food coloring, ending up with green filet of sole, blue mashed potatoes, orange cauliflower, and pink milk. We could hardly contain our excitement as we watched her dive into her dinner. At first, she seemed undaunted, but a few bites in, she put down her fork and admitted the rainbow hues had killed her appetite. We shrieked with glee. We won!

Once upon a time, we considered a plate sufficiently decorated with just a sprig of parsley or dusting of paprika. Today, the plates coming out of upscale restaurant kitchens are works of art. The chef has chosen foods in a variety of colors and textures and given the design plenty of white space around it. The fancier the restaurant, the more artful the presentation of each dish—also the smaller the servings, and the higher the price.

The beauty of the plate fills our eyes, and I believe that helps us feel satisfied with less. Here are some ways to add color and interest to your plates:

- My example descriptions aren't exactly appetizing, but I hope you get the idea. Plate #1: Lamb chop (brown C-shape), peas (little green balls), mashed potato (white blob). Plate #2: Salmon fillet (orange wedge), broccoli (green trees), rice (small white pellets).
- Although the foods in a stir fry are not in distinct positions on the plate, they combine a lot of bright colors and textures in one dish next to (or perched on top of) white rice.
- If supper is a bowl of chili or stew—normally a big heap of brown lumps—add a dollop of sour cream, some red salsa, or chopped green onions. Voilà!

Besides beauty, the other advantage of a varied plate is that it reduces palate boredom. By that I mean you can take a bite or two of one food, then a bite or two of the next one, and so on, eating your way around the plate. In this manner, you keep your senses awake.

Test this for yourself. Instead of "eating around the plate," eat the entire serving of one food—the protein, the vegetable, or the starch—without switching. As you work your way through, say, the mashed potatoes, you'll notice the first couple of bites are tastier than the last ones because your senses have gotten lazy and bored. In psychology, this diminished pleasure by repetition is known as *hedonic adaptation*. (See chapter 17, "Rate Your Food.")

The final perk of beautifying your plate is that it takes time and it takes thought. You have the opportunity to *pause* and appreciate the nourishing gift of food. In arranging the foods in a pleasing manner, you remind yourself, "I deserve this beauty, and I'm grateful for it." You and whomever else you're feeding will feel the love expressed in this extra effort.

Practice: As an act of devotion, give yourself the gift of an artful plate. As you plan your next meal, consider colors and textures and how they could be arranged on the plate. Do you have a particular plate that would show off your color choices? Channel your inner artist (you have one, I promise) and arrange the foods in a way that pleases your eye. Pluck a flower from the yard or that sprig of parsley, or even one of your children's action figures to enliven the plate. Have fun. Bon appétit.

Pause for Gratitude

As much as I claimed to love food, before creating Thin Within I ate on autopilot most of the time, paying attention to how it tasted only when it was terrible or really fantastic. It's eggs. It's spinach. It's a peanut butter and jelly sandwich. It's a Hershey's Kiss. It's salad. It's lasagna. It's vanilla ice cream. OK, fine—been there, done that. Next?

I had been so unappreciative of the edible blessings before me every day!

To remedy this injustice, I began a new practice: pausing to invite gratitude to join me at the table. I encourage you to try it. It doesn't matter what the food is. Perhaps you cooked it, perhaps someone else did. Perhaps you have no idea who prepared it, because it's a bag of chips, a Snickers bar, or a frozen dinner you just thawed. Doesn't matter. You are so fortunate not to go hungry, as so many people do all over the world.

Gratitude reminds us that we are connected to and dependent upon everything and everyone. You do not need to be religious to see food as a blessing. If you are, you may already have prayers you say before a meal. I like to use this brief pause to imagine all the hands that brought the food to me, as well as the sun, rain, and soil that nurtured it.

Practice: Gratitude break. It's time to eat. Stop and take three deep calming breaths, and acknowledge the food in front of you. Your expression of gratitude will be different every time, depending on the food and your mood. Some people say a prayer; others make up words on the spot. Whatever works for you.

Here's an example of what I said to my dinner the other night:

> *I am so grateful for this meal and for all that had to come together to bring it to me. (Here I visualized the amber waves of grain, the lambs grazing in the meadow, the farmworker picking the tomatoes—romanticizing the scenes, I know, but it felt loving.) I honor the labor of those who nurtured this food, harvested its abundance, and brought it to the supermarket where I bought it. (Here I visualized the truck drivers, shelf stockers, and cashiers.) May this meal nourish me in body and spirit that I may serve the well-being of all.*

Needless to say, this is easier to imagine when the food is simple and natural. If you see a bunch of strange chemical names on the food label, who do you thank—some robot in an artificial flavor factory in New Jersey? Should you be seeking out less processed foods?

• • • • • REMEMBER THIS • • • • •

- The soil, sun, rain, and many hands came together to bring you this food.
- How fortunate you are not to go hungry!
- Gratitude helps us transcend our petty concerns and grounds us in the present moment, the only moment we have.

24

Breaking the Spell

"True thins" do not imbue food with special powers. They eat to live and they enjoy eating, but they don't live to eat. They're not attached to food. They're not enchanted or possessed by it. Food is functional, even pleasurable, but it doesn't pulse with irresistible magnetic energy.

Such detached attitudes toward food were foreign to me, a person who looked slim enough on the outside but harbored a bottomless pig on the inside. I realized I'd given food way too much power when I had to restrain myself from diving into Carol's garbage can for her half-eaten piece of pie. Food had become such an extension of myself that I knew I'd make no progress until I could break its spell.

In fairy tales, magic spells are broken when the hero says the secret incantation or performs some kind of ritual. I knew no incantations, but in a flash, I knew exactly what the ritual had to be. A sacrifice.

A sacrifice to the gods of the garbage can.

Our stainless-steel garbage can became the holy shrine into which I would practice making my ritual sacrifices. Like putting my toe into the chilly Atlantic waters of my childhood, then gradually tiptoeing up to my knees before taking the plunge, I eased myself into this new spiritual practice.

First, I made offerings of crusts and uneaten peas from the kids' plates.

You're probably wondering, How hard can that be? Trust me, it was hard. Even though the kids' leftovers were not *my* leftovers, any food near me *could be mine*, which was as good as believing it *was* mine. So discarding it proved more challenging than a rational person might imagine. I'd become accustomed to popping these unappetizing morsels into my own mouth. Fortunately, the wiser part of my brain, teeny tiny as it was in those early days, recognized that these bits weren't anything I really wanted to eat, so my first sacrificial step took just two days to master.

Once my symbolic toes were wet, I moved up to my symbolic knees. Next level sacrifice: I would set aside the last bite of each food on my own plate and scrape it into the garbage can's waiting maw, no matter how tasty it was or how hungry I might still feel. I tossed my head with studied nonchalance like it was no big deal. In my food diary I could write *1 serving of salmon minus 1 bite, 1 serving of rice pilaf minus 1 bite*, etc. That felt good.

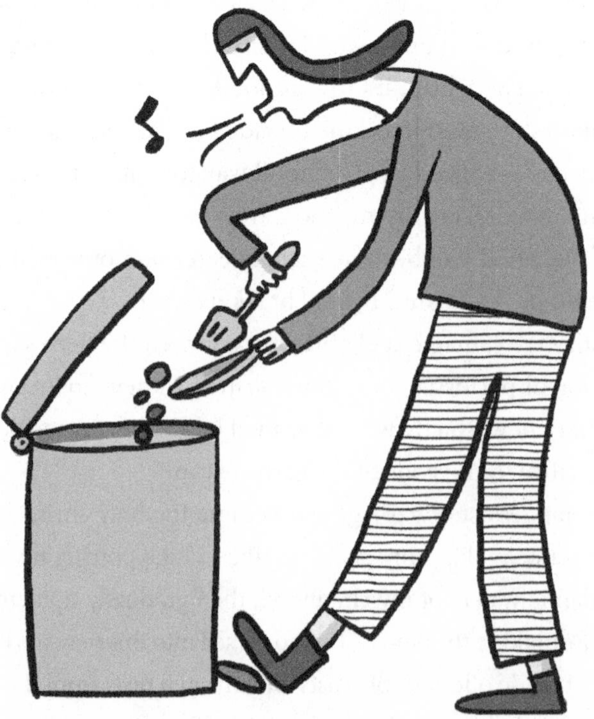

It occurred to me that I shared something in common with a hoarder. Both of us identify with things and invest extra meaning in them. We tell ourselves stories about why this thing is essential and what it represents:

I might need it someday (I might get hungry later).

It belonged to a special person (Grandma cooked it).

It reminds me of a happy time (cake = my eighth birthday party).

It is part of a collection (who eats eggs without bacon or toast?).

It is rare and unique (I may never get to eat chocolate fondue again).

On and on, story after story. To let food go meant losing a crucial part of myself.

Up to my symbolic hips now. I would make my sacrifices a game where I pitched the leftovers from increasing distances, like a free throw in basketball. This messy, irreverent act broke the spell; it lightened my spirits and reminded me that I had more power than my food. After an unusually generous offering of spaghetti from Heather's plate splatted itself down the side of the can, I had to scale back the drama, satisfying though it was for a moment. I didn't want to give the kids any (more) bad ideas.

With daily practice it became easier to detach myself from the food on my plate. It was with great smugness that I also resigned from the Clean Plate Club.

Practice: Pitch it. At every meal, leave a small part of the food on your plate to scrape into the sacrificial garbage can—*especially something that you like.* Notice where in your body you feel grabby as you do this, and what thoughts and emotions come up for you. Don't let some other family member clear your plate; you must do it yourself. You need to be present to the experience of letting that shit go. Write about these experiences in your notebook. You are reclaiming your power. Yay, you!

In the next chapter you will have an experience of how attraction and aversion feels in your body.

• • • • • REMEMBER THIS • • • • •

- Food is not love. It is not your mother. It is not your enemy either. Food is food.
- Just as you were the one who gave food a special power, you can release yourself from its grasp.

25

Body Break II: Rev Up Your Ch'i

Energy in Chinese medicine, feng shui, and the Asian martial arts is called ch'i. It's the vital life force moving through you all the time—sometimes it flows unimpeded and sometimes it is sluggish. Sluggish ch'i casts a deadening pall on your mood and motivation. So, let's wake it up. I recommend you do all six steps of the practice below, but if you only have time for the first three, that's better than doing nothing. However, the entire sequence takes less than five minutes once you figure it out.

Repeat this as many times a day as needed to enliven your energy and remind yourself that you have a body.

Practice: Rev up your ch'i.

1. **Check in.** Stand up and find a space where you can move your arms without hitting anything. Close your eyes for a moment and notice whether you can sense energy running through you. You may or may not notice anything. That's fine. Now inhale and exhale deeply three times. Open your eyes.
2. **Shake it out.** Remember the hokey pokey? This is a version of that. One at a time shake out each leg, then rotate and wiggle each ankle. Now shake and flap your arms until you feel kind of tingly. Loosely flap your hands, then open and close your fists several times. If you can, twist from side to side a few times with your arms slapping loosely against you like empty coat sleeves. Roll your shoulders up, back and down, then reverse. Reach up and give your scalp a quick scritch, like a (dry) shampoo.

3. **Stretch.** Roll your head gently from side to side, then forward and back to release your overworked neck muscles. Next, reach one arm as high up as you can while simultaneously reaching the other arm as far down as you can. You are connecting the energy between heaven and earth. Repeat on the other side. Would some other stretch also feel good now? Do that.
4. **Experience attraction and aversion.** The purpose of this step is to help you recognize, in a physical way, your attraction to food and aversion to letting it go to waste. Lift your arms shoulder height in front of you, and imagine you're holding a taut elastic rope in each fist. Let your breath out. Now, as you inhale, pull those ropes in toward you, feeling the resistance. Open your fists and, as you exhale loudly, push your hands away from you as if you were shutting a very heavy door. Repeat twice more, imagining as you do, that you are stronger than the magnetic energy of food.
5. **Clear any remaining cobwebs from your head.** Cover your ears with your hands, then move them a couple of inches out on each side. Now imagine they're propelling the wheels on a train as you rotate them forward in circles about foot in diameter. Does your scalp begin to prickle? If not, run your fingers through your hair and give your scalp a scritch-scritch.
6. **Repeat Step 1, the check-in.** Do you feel any different?

• • • • • REMEMBER THIS • • • • •

- Movement is the body's love language.
- When energy flows in the body, it brings flow to the mind.

26

Positive Programming

Begin to be now what you will be hereafter.
Man can alter his life by altering his thinking.
—William James

When you took yourself through the "The Wall Comes Down" meditation, you constructed and destroyed this barrier and let your better self out. (If you ignored the meditation… well, you're spectating, not participating.)

Your goal-mindset is still wobbly—like a baby learning to walk. Also, like a baby, your goal-mindset will benefit from some encouragement and a kindly guiding hand. Meanwhile, that old negative programming is fighting tooth and tongue for survival. It screams in desperation, "Who are you kidding! You'll never succeed!" You would never speak like that to someone you loved, would you?

When we're unable to imagine an alternative future, we talk ourselves into believing we're doomed to repeat the failures of the past, thus creating a future that does just that. What we believe determines our actions, which determines our outcomes. (How many ways can I repeat this point?)

You've done your best to set fat-mindset aside, but now what? If you don't put something in the sinkhole that had been occupied by your negative self-talk, those thoughts will rush back in to fill the void. Since you're already constantly talking to yourself, why not turn that self-talk into a practice of saying positive, encouraging things to yourself about your new identity? As everyone's mom used to say to us, "Dear, you catch more flies with honey than with vinegar."

Affirmations

Affirmations are positive statements that remind you of your strengths, intentions, and best qualities. These are assertions that are stated unequivocally and with confidence. They're always stated in the present tense, as if they are *a reality* right now.

Affirmations were popularized by Shakti Gawain's perennial bestseller, *Creative Visualization*. She expanded the technique of guided meditation by using frequently repeated affirmative statements to strengthen your visions and bring them into being. You'll like them if you're a fan of "the law of attraction."

Although you may not have been aware of it, you've probably been using affirmations all along, in areas of your life where the results were apparent. You may have told yourself things like, *I am a good teacher, I am a skillful artist, I'm a thoughtful neighbor.* And you are. Now we're going to expand your affirmative reach into the area of weight mastery.

Once I had a clear image of my inner ideal self, I created a series of affirmations to replace my negative self-talk. True confession: at first I found them hokey, but they turned out to be so effective, we incorporated them into our Thin Within classes, where participants used them as examples to craft their own. One gal in our workshop, Alva B., set her affirmations to the cowboy song, "The Streets of Laredo," so she could sing them to herself as she took her daily walk:

I am a hundred and twenty-pound person
And I only eat what that person would eat.
So each little taste bud is carefully tasting.
They know I am with them each morsel I eat.

I sit at my table, not troubled nor fretting.
I look at my food and I like what I see.
Each mouthful I chew with great love and attention
But if I don't like it, it won't become me.

Whenever I'm hungry, I eat what my soul craves.
I eat till I'm full, not a tiny bite more.
This is no diet—it's just pure excitement.
For food is a friend. Could you ask for much more?

In the following meditation I share some affirmations that bolstered my goal mindset. You can listen to this recording often. However, it's much more powerful to create your own affirmations, so they express your particular needs in your own words.

Set aside several minutes where you won't be disturbed and have your notebook nearby so you can take notes when we're done. Your job is to let the images and words wash over you.

Important! Don't worry if you find yourself arguing with every phrase. That's your resistance talking. We'll deal with that in the next part of the book. As Martin Luther King Jr. said, "Take the first step in faith. You don't have to see the whole staircase."

Guided Meditation: Affirming Your Ideal-Sized Self. After you listen, you'll see my sample affirmations below.

Prompt: Write *at least* ten affirmations in your own wording. They can be the same as any I just read, or entirely different. The one rule: they must be positive and they must be stated in the present tense, as if they are a reality *right now*. I offer mine below as a starting place, but please alter them to better suit your needs and preferences. If you want to write your own song, so much the better.

Practice: Daily Affirmations. Add to your affirmation list every day. You can read them to yourself, write them repeatedly in your notebook, record them as a voice memo on your phone for playback several times a day, or any combination of these. They can help you create a positive frame for the day ahead if you repeat them to yourselves on waking in the morning. My examples, as I recorded them on the guided meditation:

I am the master of my eating.
I'm at peace with food and free of its spells.
I slowly savor my food, grateful for the pleasure it brings.
I am attracted to foods that improve my health.
I eat when I'm sitting down in a calm environment.
I eat only when I'm physically hungry.
I recognize when I've eaten just enough and simply stop eating.
I feel good about stopping before I'm full.
I eat selectively, only those foods that appeal to me.
I love to awaken my palate with new foods and new cuisines.
I enjoy the power of leaving food on my plate.
I am stronger than a bag of potato chips, more powerful than fudge.
At parties I focus on getting to know other people, not the buffet.
I can say "No, thank you," without feeling the least bit guilty.
I can throw food away without pangs of attachment.
I can leave my tired excuses behind.
I appreciate this miraculous body I've been given.
I treat my body with love and compassion.
I'm the only me in the whole world, so I carry myself with pride.
I have many skillful ways to deal with my feelings besides eating.
I am the master of my eating.
I'm at peace with food and my body.

• • • • • REMEMBER THIS • • • • •

- To affirm is to assert a goal *as a present fact.*
- When you affirm your positive qualities, you bolster your ability to act more positively. In turn, you'll get more positive results. Frequent repetition imbeds these qualities in your brain and begins to crowd out that nagging negativity.

PART FIVE
Traps, Tricks, and Treats

You are well on your way. Nevertheless, like on any proper hero's journey, there will be dragons, or pirates, or potluck parties waiting to ambush you. And snacks. Ah, snacks. We look at how to turn these obstacles into opportunities for learning. Do not be discouraged. This is a herky-jerky process of three steps forward and one step back. Your job is to keep going. It is a life practice.

27

Teaser or Pleaser? SuperTool #5

I can resist anything, except temptation.
—Oscar Wilde

You can't always control your circumstances, but you can control your response. One way to gain more control over your responses is to distinguish between something that teases you into an action that your wiser self knows won't be satisfying, and something that will both please and satisfy you. I call these Teasers and Pleasers.

This novel way of classifying foods has nothing to do with nutritional value and everything to do with the satisfaction you get out of eating.

Teasers. A Teaser is a food that snares you with its bony beckoning finger as you pass it on the counter, open the snack drawer, smell it in the movie theater, or see it advertised on TV. It's convenient and requires little thought or effort to pop into your mouth. You may not be hungry when you see it, and you may not even really like it, but once you see it, you immediately go into wanting mode. Before you know it, you've succumbed to its teasing presence. Unfortunately, it doesn't fill that empty wanting place. In the world of behavioral science, a Teaser is a kind of trigger because it's a cue to act out a habitual behavior. (Remember fat machinery in chapter 13?)

We are surrounded by Teasers every day (not just the food kind), and their easy ubiquity makes them hard to resist. In regards to eating, there are two kinds of Teasers—one is set off by a sensory cue and the other by the *shoulds* in your belief system.

Teaser examples set off by sensory triggers (sight, smell, sound):

- The bowl of chips on the coffee table (sight)
- The cheap candies in the dish on the receptionist's desk (sight)
- The fancy dessert the waiter describes in glowing terms (sound and maybe sight)
- The odors of Cinnabon at the shopping mall (smell)
- The crunching of popcorn in the movie theater (sound and smell)

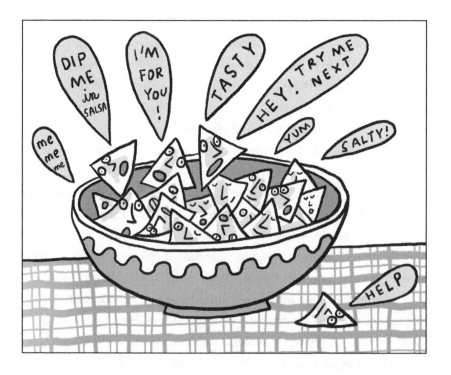

Teaser examples set off by the *shoulds* in your belief system

- The last bites on your plate after you're already full (a Clean Plate Club *should*)

- The kale salad you know is good for you, but you don't much like kale (a nutritional *should*)
- The carrots, celery, or sugarless cookies you eat instead of the scone you really want (a diet-mind *should*)

Pleasers. A Pleaser begins with a food image in your mind. It's very specific—prepared in a particular way or served just so. It's probably not in front of you when it comes to mind, and it may take some effort to get or create it. It may only be available in a certain season (tree-ripened peaches) or location (Maine lobster roll). When you do get it… ahhhh! It was worth the wait and the trouble. A Pleaser ends the quest for satisfaction. You want nothing more. If the Japanese clutter-clearing queen, Marie Kondo, were watching, she would note that your Pleaser "sparks joy." Here are a few of mine:

- The dense butterscotch pudding at Portland's Irving Street Kitchen
- Heirloom tomatoes still warm from the garden, sprinkled with crunchy salt
- Mom's broiled shrimp in garlic butter
- Grilled Japanese eggplant, served with a sesame oil sauce
- Blackberry cobbler with whipped cream

Pleasers will change with your mood or situation. They can be weird combinations that only you would find appealing. I once had a thing for an onion sandwich: two pieces of buttered toast, a thick slice of Vidalia onion and lots of ketchup. It was a passion no one else shared. (Nor did anyone want me near afterwards.)

The mere act of identifying a food as a Teaser or Pleaser goes a long way toward choosing the best response.

Is It a Teaser or a Pleaser?

Discernment between Teasers and Pleasers requires a certain amount of self-knowledge and conscious deliberation. This is impossible if you're not paying attention. During my time teaching Thin Within, we asked participants to bring their favorite snack for one of our taste-testing exercises. Most were surprised to discover that their snack was a Teaser, not a Pleaser. When experienced slowly in the present moment, it often didn't live up to their expectations.

They also realized that almost every food considered to be "diet food" was a Teaser—not that it was inherently unpleasing, but it had been *prescribed*, not *chosen*. Case in point, cottage cheese, a high-protein *should* that used to be a popular diet food. Back in my dieting days, I ate a LOT of cottage cheese in hopes it would melt away my fat, like it did for the folks in the magazine articles. Even after I'd filled up on it, I usually found myself rummaging through the fridge looking for a little something more—something that would be *satisfying*.

Utilitarian foods. At first Marie Kondo was pretty hardcore about the stuff her clutter-clearing clients should keep—only those things that "sparked joy." Then she got pushback from readers who asked questions like, "Well, what about my vacuum cleaner? My kitchen table? My toaster oven? These don't give me a tingle of joy, but they do the job and I need them." She had to acknowledge that it's OK to keep certain things around for simple utilitarian purposes.

Much of what we eat on a daily basis *is* utilitarian—perfectly good food that does the job of nourishing us. Meat and potatoes, as it were. Not every bite will spark joy or hit your Pleaser sweet spot. Nevertheless, it's important to be aware of the danger of Teasers and to seek more Pleasers when you can.

Teasers are everywhere, in all aspects of our lives, not only in edible form. Think about shopping for clothes. You see a *Sale!* sign on the boutique door and WOW! Two shirts for the price of one! You don't need any more shirts, but you'd be crazy to pass up such a deal, so you plunk down your money, delighted with your shopping skill. Two years later, those two shirts still hang unworn in your closet, tags dangling. Sad to say, most sales (of whatever) are glorified Teasers.

Invitations can also be Teasers. The invitation shows up in your inbox. You look on your calendar and see, "Yup, I'm free that night," so you RSVP that you'll be there, even though you hardly know the host. Instead, test your faculties of discernment. Before opening your calendar, ask yourself a few questions. Would this particular event be fun or helpful? Am I only accepting because I'm afraid I'll miss out on something? It is OK to politely decline.

Dessert-pushing waiters are Teasers. I once had trouble resisting them until I developed a new strategy. As I slowly read the dessert menu, I use my eyes and my imagination to taste each tempting Teaser one by one down the list. This mental trick can be quite filling. Then I tell the ever hopeful waiter, "Alas, I am full." If one of those rejected desserts continues to haunt me, I can always return to the restaurant a few days later and order just that dessert.

Recognize your opportunity costs. If you want to lose or maintain your weight, there's a finite amount of calories you can consume in a day without penalty. If you eat a lot of chips, then you have no caloric room or space for the pork chop. Likewise you have a finite amount of time and energy. If you spend the evening watching TV, you can't spend the evening reading to your children. Now that you understand the difference between Teasers and Pleasers, consider the power of applying your discernment to other areas of your life:

- Those acquaintances you keep hanging out with out of habit, despite no longer having much in common? Is it time to make new friends?
- That cousin you haven't spoken to in a couple of years but always makes you laugh and feel appreciated? Why not give him a call and find a way to reconnect?

- Do you participate in certain activities that are no longer fulfilling, but you still do them out of obligation? Obliged to whom? Why?
- You've always wanted to visit Paris, but spend your free time on social media. Why not practice your French or learn about French history instead?

You get the idea. You have many choices available to you—what will you do?

✏📖 **Prompt: My Teasers and Pleasers.** In your notebook create two lists, one titled "Teasers" and the other, "Pleasers." Start by listing foods, then branch out to activities, people, whatever. These are in the moment, changeable. As you become more skillful at discerning one from the other, do include more Pleasers in your life. You deserve to have those joyful sparks.

• • • • • REMEMBER THIS • • • • •

- A Teaser is a two-for-one deal where you didn't really even need or want one.
- A Pleaser—in food and in life—is worth the wait or the work to get it.

28

Speaking of Cottage Cheese

Cottage cheese, broken down into its simplest form, is milk that has been curdled to mimic the cellulite its consumption is meant to banish.
—Elsie Love

One reason to carry your notebook with you at all times is that you never know when something will set off a cascade of emotions. Capturing it on the page right then and there can open the door to an important realization.

Soon after I taught my first Thin Within session on fat machinery, I found myself standing in front of the open refrigerator, looking for something—*anything* besides what I was supposed to be doing, like writing down what I'd teach in the next session.

My eye landed on the ever-present container of cottage cheese. Years earlier, I had read in a women's magazine that cottage cheese was the world's fastest fat burner. If memory serves, I was supposed to eat it three times a day, then through the miracle of ketosis my fat would just blow away with each exhalation. Like all the diets I'd tried and abandoned back then, the cottage cheese diet never lasted more than 24 hours. Nevertheless, I was still clutching the belief that cottage cheese *could* be the answer, so I always kept some on hand. Because I didn't really like it, the contents of the ignored container often went funky, the white curds turning slimy orange around the edges.

That day, when I caught sight of the cottage cheese, I felt my face get hot with anger. *What was going on?* I realized the very existence of cottage cheese enraged me. I grabbed my notebook and scribbled my thoughts as they tumbled out of my brain. [NB: I have (mostly) avoided using swear words in this book, even though I'm quite fond of them in my off-the-page life. If you're offended by the F-word (the four-letter one), you can skip this section, although you'll miss a rip-roaring cathartic experience you might sometime want to try for yourself.]

May 20. So much food in the fridge! I feel the urge to eat it or cook it all up RIGHT NOW. If I don't eat it or cook it up RIGHT NOW it may SPOIL.

Letting cottage cheese spoil is bad.

Letting cottage cheese spoil is good.

Letting cottage cheese spoil is funny.

Letting cottage cheese spoil costs 50 cents.

Letting cottage cheese spoil might be worth it.

Letting the whole fucking fridge spoil might be worth it.

I don't want the cottage cheese.

Cottage cheese fucking RUNS me.

Wasting food runs me.

FUCK the cottage cheese!

FUCK the pumpkin puree.

FUCK the leftover noodles parmesan.

Fuck the 7 fish sticks, the 4 tired tortillas, the All-Bran muffins.

And fuck the boring meat loaf, the limp carrots, the tofu.

Not to mention the alfalfa sprouts, the cabbage, the potatoes.

And the oats, dry milk, brown sugar.

The jam, the apples, the jar of peanut butter.

Definitely fuck the peanut butter...

The words tumbled out as fast as I could write. I realized I could name every scrap of food in the kitchen without opening a single cupboard. I had no idea my emotions ran so deep. Was it about the food, or about its spell on me? It was both. I knew I had a thing about wasting food, which often fueled extreme bursts of creative cooking, but I'd been unaware how *compelled* I was to make use of *everything*. After I closed my notebook, some previously unnoticed tension inside me relaxed, like after good sex.

✏📖 **Prompt: Emotion dump.** The next time you find yourself with strong feelings, either for or against some food, get out your notebook and let 'er rip onto the page. It could be random phrases, a poem, a drawing, snippets of a memory. Have fun!

A year after the cottage cheese incident, I attended a conference on time management in San Francisco because I was intrigued by the link between procrastination and eating. The keynote speaker was the time management guru of the early 1970s, Alan Lakein, author of the bestseller, *How to Get Control of Your Time and Your Life*. His advice seems like common wisdom nowadays, but it was new to me: set measurable goals for yourself, create action steps toward them, and prioritize those steps—A,B, and C. If I recall, A = must do, B = should do, C = do only if you've got time to spare.

After Lakein delivered his talk, I shared with him how helpful I'd found his book. It was just before lunch, and he asked me to join him. Although there were many tasty offerings on the Sheraton Palace menu, he ordered the cottage cheese plate with fruit. I don't recall what I ordered, but you can be sure it wasn't cottage cheese. He did most of the talking, for which I was grateful, because I was watching this slim man eat.

In the center of his plate was a round scoop of cottage cheese, ringed by two canned apricot halves and three half-slices of pineapple, topped with a maraschino cherry. Straightaway, he plucked off the cherry and popped it into his mouth, then he methodically worked his way around the fruits on the perimeter—first the pineapple, then the apricot halves. Finally, he took two bites of the cottage cheese. At that point, he pushed his plate back. "Dammit!" he exclaimed, patting his stomach. "My 'A' priority was the protein in the cottage cheese, but I got sidetracked by the fruit, which was only a 'C', and now I'm full!"

I had to laugh at how this particular true-thin's mind worked. In Lakein's time-management approach to life, food had been reduced to a set of A, B, and C priorities.

To this day, I cannot see "Cottage Cheese Plate" on a menu without thinking of my lunch with Lakein. Nor have I bought a single tub of those white curds since I scribbled my rant.

• • • • • REMEMBER THIS • • • • •

- Life lessons are everywhere. So is inspiration.
- Enjoy the ride.

29

Your Kitchen: Friend or Foe

If you learned nothing else during your dieting days, you realized that it's hard to continually exercise your willpower. It's much easier if you set up your environment so that willpower is unnecessary. As James Clear (author of *Atomic Habits*, one of the three best books on habit change I've ever read—see Appendix C) suggests, "You don't have to be the victim of your environment. You can also be the architect of it."

During the weeks when I recorded everything I ate, it became readily apparent that my kitchen was hazardous to my health—not because the food it contained wasn't nutritious, but because that's where the food lived, and I spent an inordinate amount of time in its proximity, exposed to its temptations. It was a non-stop Teaser.

Monkey see, monkey eat. Or maybe "chicken see, chicken eat." Years ago, I read a study about the eating behavior of chickens. As I recall, the researchers put a couple of chickens in a large coop and placed a dish of grain in the middle of the enclosure. The chickens ate until they were satisfied, then wandered off to scratch and cluck. Then the researchers placed a new chicken in the coop. She spotted the grain dish and began to eat. As soon as the original chickens saw her eating, they returned to the dish and ate more. When sated, all three wandered off. Several times more the researchers added a new chicken, and each time the incumbent chickens joined her to eat yet again. The original chickens must have been stuffed to the beak!

The dismal truth: many of us behave like one of those chickens, with a propensity to eat every time we see food, whether or not we're hungry. How can we prevent those conditioned responses?

In my case, the refrigerator lurked right beside the back door, waiting to snag my attention. Many times a day, especially if I was bored, I'd have to check it out. What was happening in there? Had anything changed since last I looked? Had the cheese gotten moldy? Were we running low on celery? Did I remember to call the dentist? Is there a God?

Whether or not the answer could be found inside the fridge (hope sprang eternal), anything was possible. Of course, every time I opened the fridge door, I ate something. The cheese tasted pretty good, actually. Another bite to make sure. Yes, we had celery, though it looked a tad limp. Did it still have crunch? A nibble to test. Oh dear, the peanut butter has somehow gotten hidden behind the jam. How much is in the jar? Mmm, peanut butter. I do love peanut butter. It's protein. Maybe put some on the celery to give it more oomph?

The kitchen counter also held a magnetic trap—"an attractive nuisance" in the parlance of the insurance industry—a big glass jar of granola, homemade by me, Super Mom! So crunchy. So very nutritious. So easy to pop the lid and reach in for a handful. And another. I bet it would be good on vanilla yogurt. Let's see, ah, there's the yogurt, behind the dill pickles. Must try.

Years later, I learned that in many Asian traditions they consider everything to be *alive—alive with meaning*. Humans are symbolic creatures, and even though we're rarely aware of it, we imbue the objects around us with meaning and stories. If we pay attention we can hear their subliminal messages.

Teaser foods are teasers because they're talking to you. Those brownies on the counter are begging to be eaten before they get stale—like in the next two minutes. Or they're whispering, *Please tidy up our crumbs.*

"You-proof" your kitchen. If you want to be a smarter chicken and prevent unwanted temptations, I recommend a kitchen detox, so it isn't a teasing saboteur. The following exercise will make you more aware of the traps. Get into a sleuthing mode and grab your notebook to record any discoveries.

✎📖 **Prompt: The kitchen walk-through.** Start with the most obvious. What's visible as you enter the room? Are there edible temptations on the countertops? Does the refrigerator have a commanding position by the door, making it hard to ignore? (I'm not suggesting a remodel, just notice it).

Open the cupboard doors where you store dry goods. Take everything out and place it all on the counter or table. What kinds of foods do you have a lot of and what kinds not much of? What gets used and what doesn't? What is easy to access, and what is more hidden? Make some notes.

Might as well wipe down the cupboard shelves before you put stuff back. Feel free to rearrange things or toss anything unused or expired.

On to the refrigerator, starting with the freezer. Once again, pull everything out and ask yourself the same questions as above. (You can defrost another time. For now, just put back what you're keeping). Make some notes, then repeat the process with the main part of the refrigerator. What kinds of foods predominate? Are there many fresh fruits and veggies? Are you big into condiments? Leftovers? How fast do foods move through? Do certain foods spoil before you get around to eating them? Again, take notes.

In general, who is your kitchen stocked for—to please children, a partner, potential guests, yourself? Is this the kitchen of someone who is health-conscious? What can you change to make your kitchen serve you better—as a cook (or non-cook, that's OK, too) and as a person who is committed to completing this "freedom project?"

Do you (and your family) eat in the kitchen in view of the stove, or in a separate dining space? If you can see additional food when you're eating, it can tease you just like it does the chickens.

One more thing. Examine your plates, bowls, glasses, and eating utensils. What is the diameter of the plates on which you usually eat? (See chapter 5.) Were you aware that spoons and forks have also gotten bigger in the past few decades, so even a single bite is now bigger?

Review your notes. Are there changes you'd like to make? Make a list and get started.

REMEMBER THIS

- Willpower is overrated. Create an environment that doesn't require it.
- A supportive environment makes weight mastery much easier.

30

Cue the Negative Pushback

When you begin affirming your positive qualities, the first thing that pops up in the mind is a healthy skepticism. It sure did for me. *Is this some kind of New Age mumbo-jumbo?*

That's your resistance talking. It says things like "You are NOT and never will be slim." Resistance doesn't want to repeat affirmations, so it declares, "I'm smarter than that." Or "I don't have the time for this foolishness."

Welcome to the negative pushback. Change is hard, especially when you're changing behaviors, beliefs, and habits you've spent a lifetime fabricating. Giving up the old ways—to make way for what? The unknown is scary.

Invariably in a Thin Within class, a participant would ask "Aren't affirmations a form of brainwashing?" Well, yes, you could say that. However, have you not been brainwashing yourself with fat-mind negativity for years?

When my friend Chérie asked, "What if the obstacle *is* the path?" she was suggesting that I needed to face my current reality, which included a great deal of negative self-talk. Instead of denying its existence, I needed to look it in the eye and begin to fight back.

Even though affirmations helped me promote my new self-image and encourage "goal-mindset" behaviors, I had to acknowledge the strength of my resistance, which manifested in the form of berating myself. Rather than let my resistance fester as I repeated my affirmations, I started writing the negative self-talk down in my notebook, where I could examine it more objectively. (It must be noted I was an extremely harsh self-critic).

Love this body? Really? Look at you! Stomach pooching out on the outside, selfish slut on the inside. Who are you to talk about perfection? Hahaha! Right now, I do not love this body. It has behaved badly and should be ashamed.

Only eating when hungry? OK, slight improvement there, but last night I saw you stuff your face with the last of the spaghetti, even though you knew you were full. (Damn tasty though; you make killer sauce.)

Treat yourself with kindness? Why? You yelled at Ethan for not finishing his breakfast—you, who tell your students it's all right to leave food on their plate—so hypocritical.

Surprisingly, as I paid attention to the voice of my resistance, the simple act of naming and noting it in my notebook caused it to deflate. Sometimes I talked out loud to that voice: *Ha! So, you're trying to con me into buying a bag of Cheetos! I see what you're doing there.* I began to feel I was reclaiming my own power.

✎📖 **Prompt: The inquiry.** After you've created and recorded your own personalized set of affirmations and listened to them a number of times, begin listening to your internal back-talk. As if you were drafting the pro and con arguments for a voters' pamphlet, write each affirmation, and next to it your arguments against, so you can see them in black and white. It is very important to not just think this through, but to actually put the thoughts down in black and white on paper.

Next, one at a time, dig into each argument. I recommend using a powerful process of inquiry that extraordinary wise woman Byron Katie, calls "The Work." When you encounter a negative thought pattern, she asks you to explore four questions:

Sample negative thought: "Nobody loves a fat woman."

Byron Katie's four questions:

1. This thought/judgment: Is it true?
2. Can you *absolutely* know that it's true?
3. How do you react when you *think* that thought [your feelings, emotions, memories of the past, fears going into the future]?
4. Who would you be without this thought? [If you were free of this thing you tell yourself, who would you be, how would you feel?]

The fifth and final step of Katie's inquiry process is to turn the thought around and consider some opposite views. Examples of a few: "Nobody *hates* a fat woman," or "Nobody loves a *thin* woman," or "*Everybody* loves a fat woman," or "*Fat women love me.*" If this process interests you, she offers free worksheets at her website, byronkatie.com. You can also watch her do The Work with a variety of people on her YouTube channel. Highly recommended.

Your explorations will take patience and perseverance. Working your way through one negative thought or judgment per day will provide you with many freeing revelations, guaranteed.

• • • • • REMEMBER THIS • • • • •

- Resistance is a force (real or imagined) tending to prevent motion or action.
- Acknowledge your arguments and let them go.

31

Mutiny on the Bounty

You can either have the results you intend,
or your reasons why not.
—Werner Erhard, The est Training

Resistance is a strong human impulse. *Push on me, and I'm going to push back.* Resistance wears many faces, and all of them are itching for a fight. Once you can identify the forces you're up against, you'll be better prepared to counteract them. To make it easier for you to recognize them, let's take a pretend sail on the high seas.

Imagine that you're the captain of a ship on a treasure hunt. Your goal is to reach the spot marked on the map with a big red X, where the treasure (your ideal-sized self) lies.

You, the captain, are the only one who knows where you're going. Unfortunately, you made some hiring mistakes and the sailors you picked turned out to be pirates, only in it for themselves. As the ship gets closer to the treasure, the rambunctious crew mutinies and locks you in the brig. The pirates fight each other for a turn at the helm, causing the ship to veer off course. Let's meet them:

The Indulger doesn't like experiencing difficult emotions or situations. When they do arise, The Indulger says, "Go ahead! You've had a hard day. You deserve a big bowl of ice cream." **The Well-Deserved (twin sister of The Indulger)** has the same response when she's been so "good" that she deserves to indulge herself in something "bad." We all need compassionate breaks, but is ice cream the best way to care for yourself?

The Perfectionist sets high standards, and anything less than 120% is not good enough. The Perfectionist says, "You only lost two pounds this week? Big deal; you're still a TON away from your goal." Or, "I don't care if you're at 30% on the hunger scale. You shouldn't eat that cookie." The Perfectionist thinks in black and white—all or nothing. You either succeed or you fail; baby steps are for wimps. The Perfectionist means well, but needs to lighten up.

The Rebel is a resister. No one can tell a Rebel what to do. "I'm a grown-up; I don't need no stinking Winning Formula. Real men can eat over the sink and answer email at the same time." In healthiest form, the Rebel is spirited, courageous and assertive, daring you to be great.

The Martyr. In an effort to get approval from others, the Martyr abdicates her power to her noble self-sacrificing image. "I'm only eating it so I won't hurt Grandma's feelings." "I'm too busy serving you to sit down." "Everyone else is eating cake; I wouldn't want to stick out." In her best form, the Martyr just wants to love and be loved, so she needs to find better ways to express this.

The Procrastinator doesn't like facing tasks, decisions or communications that might be difficult. Sometimes the difficult thing is postponed only briefly, using fat-mind's favorite avoidance tactic, *the snack*. (Snacking is such a common issue for the weight warrior it deserves a chapter of its own, which is coming right up.) Sometimes the difficult thing—like beginning a diet or exercise program—is so daunting that the Procrastinator pulls a *tomorrow* tactic. "The hell with it today; I'll start tomorrow." Alas, you'll eventually have to do that thing.

The Willing Victim ties herself to the train tracks, then gets all upset when she gets run over. The Willing Victim engineers circumstances that prove irresistible—keeping ice cream in the freezer, asking the waiter to show her the dessert tray, offering to bake her favorite chocolate chip cookies for an event where everyone is diabetic. It's a way of *arranging to fail.* The best way to foil the Willing Victim is to recognize and laugh at her wily ways.

The Ostrich sticks her head in the sand so she won't see what she's doing. Cookie batter licked off the mixer beaters doesn't count as eating. Nor does scarfing down stray cake crumbs or making certain the leftover macs 'n' cheese casserole has the straightest of edges. Acknowledging the reality of these crumbs by recording them in your notebook wakes you up to their frequency.

Who's the captain here? We have so many ways to sabotage ourselves. And they're all stories, excuses, reasons, loopholes, get out of jail cards. The good news is that when you slow down and center yourself in the present moment you can hear these saboteurs trying to take over—and once you recognize their voices and their devilish messages, you have a conscious choice. "Oh you again! You're trying to blow me off course, but I AM THE CAPTAIN of this ship, so get lost!"

✎📖 **Prompt: Your inner pirate(s).** Imagine yourself as each one of these characters, *one by one.* You may have a particular role that is your default, or maybe you're so versatile you've played each one. In your notebook, write down how you act out each of these pirate roles—the stories and excuses you use to pull your ship off course. Then, for each of your inner pirates, imagine other responses that better support your goals. Write them down, the better to recognize their subversive games.

• • • • • REMEMBER THIS • • • • •

- You are the captain and *you* are in charge.
- If you have results, you won't need excuses.

32

Snack Attack

Several days and many snacks later,
I finally figured out what was really bugging me.
—Kate R., Thin Within participant

As I sit at my computer writing this book about mindful eating behaviors and all the ways we sabotage ourselves, I often feel stuck. *Gahhh! This is hard work,* I say to myself. *What's the best way to express this concept? How could I describe this process in a more compelling manner? What are the negative messages I still lay on myself?*

Then the sneaky voice of the **Well-Deserved** interrupts. *Joy, you've worked so hard. How 'bout a little snack?* (Yeah, that voice is still alive and kicking in me, though I rarely succumb to it.)

Snacks are a perfect diversionary tactic. They're the readily available all-purpose bandage for distracting ourselves from the uncomfortable moments in our day—boredom, confusion, fatigue, anxiety, *emotions.* A snack buys us a little time or distance from discomfort until we feel more ready to tackle whatever we're trying to avoid.

Snacks are the Teasers that travel quickly from our lips to our hips. If you could eliminate your snacking habit, it's likely you would not only lose weight, you'd also be more self-aware and productive.

Public health researchers believe that our country's obesity epidemic is directly related to the proliferation of snack foods, most of which are high in fat, sugar, and salt and low in nutrient density. In nutrition lingo, they're called "empty calories."

It's human to want to avoid discomfort. The frequency with which we reach for "a little something to eat" is uniquely American. Snacks aren't the only Band-Aid in the avoidance toolbox; we also check our email, look up something on the internet, trim our fingernails, call a friend, stand up and stretch, make a cup of tea.

Unfortunately, unlike checking email, eating a snack is a strategy with caloric consequences. After you apply a snack Band-Aid, whatever discomfort you were avoiding still remains, and now those calories are stuck on your body.

What about after-dinner snacks? In the evening, you may not be avoiding discomfort; you simply got tired of being mindful. You've moved into **The Indulger's** territory *(I deserve it; it's been a hard day)*. A snack bowl/bag/box has somehow found its way onto your coffee table where it waits for you to get distracted by the TV. While you're caught up in the drama, that hand attached to the end of your arm sidles into the bowl, feels around for a small handful, and before you know it, that wily hand has popped the snack into your mouth. Hello, **Willing Victim.**

Your mouth is delighted: salt, fat, crunch! What more could a mouth want? More—that's what—and the snack manufacturer designed it that way. Your mouth knows that you're too distracted to notice your hand diving in for a refill. And another and another. At some point you come to your senses (a commercial? your hand comes up empty? a sharp nudge in the ribs from your partner who knows you want to lose weight?). Oops. The snack won again.

Because snacks are such a handy procrastination and emotional cover-up tool, the following three exercises can be life-changing: tracking your snack habit, taste testing your favorite snack, and abstaining from snacks for a week.

✎📖 **Prompt: My Moods and My Snacks.** If you're a frequent snacker, do the following notebook exercise to chart them. Draw four columns, and title them: State of Mind, Situation, Go-To Snack, What I Could Do Instead. Down the left side of the page, copy the "State of Mind" list, and then fill in the rest of the form. Notice any patterns?

My Moods and My Snacks

State of Mind	Example of Situation	My Go-To Snack	What I Could Do Instead
Overwhelmed			
Bored			
Tired			
Anxious, Worried			
Angry			
Procrastinating			
Indecision			
Lonely, Sad, Depressed			
Watching TV/Movies			
At Work			
Driving			
Happy, Content			
?			
?			

Observations at the end of the day:

Practice: A week watching yourself snack. Mindfulness is the key to this experiment. As you find yourself reaching for a snack, enlist your curiosity. Notice and name the physical and/or mental discomfort you're experiencing that you're hoping the snack will relieve. **Eat the snack**, then once again notice and name your physical sensations and the thoughts going through your mind. Then ask yourself: **did the snack actually work as you'd hoped?** Do this for a week.

Practice: A week without snacks. You tell yourself, "But I need a break." I'm not saying you don't. Breaks are good. But for this week, *it will not be a food break*, unless you have a medical condition that requires frequent eating. For this exercise, even carrot sticks or apple slices count as a snack. Water is OK. Maybe a cup of tea.

Have your notebook handy, so when the brilliant "a snack will help" idea pops into your head, you can write down what's going on. Note the sensations that make you think a snack would help. What happened just before you had the snack idea? Are you feeling stuck? Bored? Tired? Confused? Avoiding something that seems difficult? If so, what is it?

As those feelings come up, observe them and acknowledge them. *Yup. I don't want to make that phone call. This problem has too many moving parts. I don't want to figure out what's for dinner. I'm too tired to think.* Stand up and take three deep breaths. Walk around the room or the block. Trim your fingernails. Breathe. Drink some water. Wait and do nothing.

If your snack problem is worst in the evening, consider that it might be a cover for loneliness, sadness, anxiety or anger. If you can, write about those feelings instead of eating. Noticing and putting them down on paper is the first step to finding real solutions.

A friend told me the most helpful thing he learned in his quit smoking class was to take a few breaths when he had the urge to smoke and say to himself, "The urge to smoke will pass, whether I smoke or not." And within a couple of minutes it would indeed pass. See if this works for your urge to snack.

Ways To Avoid the Snack Attack

- Don't buy snacks you find hard to resist. But if you do, "because my partner can't live without Cheetos..." Uh-huh. Sure. (**Willing Victim?**) Read on.

- Don't bring out snacks if you know you'll be distracted—and definitely don't bring out the entire container. A handful on a small plate is plenty.
- If you insist on TV snacking *and you like* carrot sticks, celery, cucumber, pickles, or apple slices, try them for mindless, harmless crunch.
- If your hands need busywork, doodle in your notebook, sort and fold the laundry as you watch, make something with your kids' PlayDoh or LEGOs.
- If you truly *love* peanuts, popcorn, or chips, give them the devoted attention they deserve! Shake out a modest serving into a lovely small bowl, turn off distractions, light a candle in homage to these treats, take a few slow, deep breaths to center yourself, and then one by one, slowly savor each salty, fatty, crunchy bite. *Ahhh!*
- Try subjecting your snack to the Pig Out Party (coming in chapter 35).

• • • • • REMEMBER THIS • • • • •

- Snacking is a Band-Aid for discomfort, not a cure.
- The discomfort revealed by *not* snacking is an opportunity for increased self-knowledge and the potential for fresh choices.
- The easiest way to avoid snacking is not to buy snack food.

33

Be Like a Rocket

Failure is life's magnifying glass.
—Niccolo Machiavelli

Right after the conclusion of my first living room Thin Within series, I took Heather and Ethan on vacation to Camp Tuolumne, the city of Berkeley's family camp near Yosemite. Despite my success at following the Winning Formula and watching my waist shrink, I approached this vacation with great trepidation. I would be at the mercy of camp food, served buffet style in bottomless quantities, three meals a day for six days. By my calculation I'd have to face **eighteen** all-you-can-eat meals in a row.

Memories resurfaced of that earlier similar experience at Camp Wyonegonic, when I packed on 25 pounds in just eight weeks. Would I be able to use the Winning Formula? As an introvert, I also worried about making small talk with strangers.

I prepared myself by visualizing the temptations ahead and considered ways to handle them. I created several new situation-appropriate affirmations. *I stay conscious of my hunger levels even in distracting circumstances. I am stronger than a pile of mashed potatoes! I am more powerful than a platter of brownies!* I repeated these to myself several times a day.

The extra physical activity at camp made me hungry, so Step #1 of the Winning Formula, *Only eat if you're hungry,* was in place. I would *center myself with a few deep breaths* (#2) before plunging into the buffet line and I would be *sitting at a table set up for eating* (#3), but after that, meals would be a test of will. How could I focus on my food or my body's signals when I was surrounded by chattering strangers?

For the first few days I kept on track. *I've* got *this!* I told myself.

On the fourth day, I had a large glass of wine before dinner, and with it my resolve dissolved. (New inner pirate identified: **The Vacationer**—*Shut up; I'm on vacation,* a subset of **The Indulger**.) I ate All The Things that evening. Since I'd already screwed up, I ate All The Things again at breakfast, and was well on my way for a repeat performance at lunch, when I happened to overhear a conversation with a guy seated near me, an astrophysicist at the Lawrence Berkeley Lab. They were discussing the current Soyuz space mission.

Space exploration mystified me, so I asked the scientist how a rocket managed to find its way straight to the moon—so far away. He told us that space navigation utilizes a system that continuously corrects the rocket's course—on course, off course, course correction; on course, off course, course correction. It's called an inertial guidance system or IGS.

It suddenly clicked. I was like a rocket on the way to the moon (my weight goal)—except for one crucial difference. When *my* ship got off course, my IGS berated me, shamed me, and warned me my goal was beyond my reach. Since total failure was imminent (**The Perfectionist** talking), I might as well keep eating.

I wanted to become more like the rocket. On course or off course, the rocket never berates or shames itself; the IGS just notes the position and makes the appropriate correction. Just because I ate half a plate of cookies, I didn't have to go "all or nothing" and finish the rest of them. Instead of adding this particular failure to my over-burdened donkey cart, I needed to acknowledge, *Yep, I ate All The Things*, and get back on course.

By dinner that night, I had regained control of my mind and my mouth. Three steps forward, one step back, three steps forward, one step back. It was a powerful lesson.

It doesn't matter how successful or unsuccessful you think you are right now. The question is whether your habits are heading in the right direction. What is your overall trajectory? As habit change expert James Clear says in *Atomic Habits*, "Your outcomes are a lagging measure of your habits—the acts you repeat and repeat. Your net worth is a lagging measure of your financial habits. Your weight is a lagging measure of your eating habits… You get what you repeat."

System failures are bound to happen. What you're doing here is creating a web of effective habits and skills, so that when you have a breakdown you can get yourself back on track *before* you pile it onto the donkey cart of failures.

When you get off course (because you will), here's the formula for course correction:

- **Acknowledge and describe what happened. Just the facts** (no interpretations or self-flagellation, please): *The hostess brought out three different cakes. She put a slice of each on my plate. I said nothing. I intended to eat one bite of each, but I finished them all.*
- **What were the immediate consequences of what you did?** *My stomach hurt. My mind was hurling insults at me. I wanted to escape.*
- **Describe what happened just before** this happened, and any emotions you may have had. *My husband made a joke about dieters. I felt embarrassed.*
- **Which inner pirate of resistance took over?** *The People Pleaser, with a touch of The Indulger.*
- **Consider what you could have done instead.** *I could have held up my hand to refuse the plate, indicating I was full. I could have passed the plate to my husband. I could have covered it with my napkin so I wouldn't have to see the temptation.*
- **What are some ways you could make yourself feel better about yourself now?** *I could remind myself that until the cake arrived, I paid attention to my hunger levels and ate modestly. I could dump my negative thoughts in my notebook, and then counteract*

them with affirmations. I could thank my body for accepting my indulgences and not firing me.

- **How could you prevent a recurrence of similar scenarios?** *I could practice some polite ways to say "no thanks."*

✏📖 **Prompt: Plan ahead for system failures.** Imagine some scenarios where you might be thrown off track. Brainstorm in your notebook. How will you prepare? Do you need to write out a couple of scripts to guide you through possible challenges? Practice them so you don't have to think in the heat of the moment.

• • • • • REMEMBER THIS • • • • •

- Separate the facts from the story, and look for the inner pirate culprit.
- Every failure presents a valuable opportunity to learn.
- A postmortem helps to prevent future detours.

34

Permission to Pig Out

The worst thing about eating a quart of ice cream is that I can't even allow myself to enjoy it.
—Jenny L., Thin Within participant

It's hard work to maintain your watch over every bite, fearing another failure, and fighting the inner pirates. They rattle their swords, "roar their terrible roars and gnash their terrible teeth" (Thank you, Maurice Sendak). Could the pirates' threats be empty after all? As Shakespeare said, "... a tale told by an idiot, full of sound and fury, signifying nothing."

What would happen if you walked out on that plank, jumped into what you believed were frigid shark-infested waters and landed instead in a warm swimming pool, complete with float toys and a guy in a tuxedo pouring you a frosty margarita?

Well, I'm giving you the opportunity to experience that scary thing you're sure will happen if you loosen the reins on your steely will: you'll eat the whole thing and be unable to stop. You'll consume the entire fudge cake, the gallon of Rocky Road ice cream, the ginormous platter of French fries, or whatever that thing is that you believe you're powerless against.

Except this time, you are going to *choose* to eat the whole thing—*on purpose and without guilt*, because *someone else* (me) told you to try it.

CONTRAINDICATIONS: Talk to your doctor before doing the Pig Out Party if you have diabetes or any other medical or mental health condition that this exercise might exacerbate. Your health is top priority.

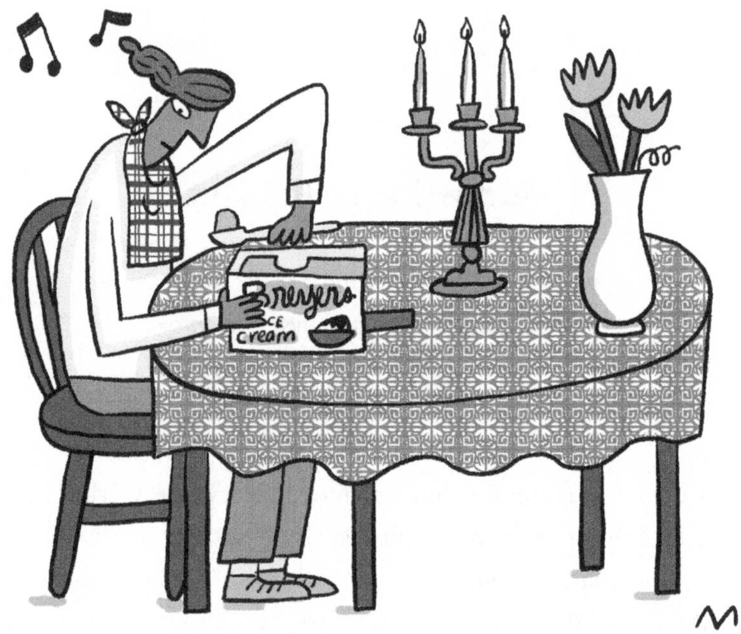

Not everyone fears they'll totally lose control, but if it worries you, here's your chance to face those fears. I hope you'll do this exercise, following the instructions below.

Prompt: Your Pig Out Party

1. Think of a food that you really like, but you try to avoid it because you're afraid that, once you got started eating it, you'd never be able to stop. It could be a standing rib roast, but more likely it's either something sweet and rich or a crunchy, salty, greasy snack food.
2. Acquire or prepare this food in a quantity that could serve at least four people.
3. Find a time when you will not be disturbed or distracted for at least half an hour, and when your internal fuel gauge is at or below 30% to give you plenty of stomach space for your treat.

4. Set up an attractive place to sit. Do you need candles? Soft music? Assemble any necessary utensils, get your notebook and pen, and place your "frenemy" (the platter of brownies, the giant bag of chips, the ice cream container or whatever your thing is) in front of you.

5. Take three centering breaths, then spend a couple of minutes examining the forbidden item closely, as if you'd never seen it before. Sniff it to discover any odors, poke it with your fingers to see how it feels. As you do, observe any physical sensations you're experiencing. Has your hunger level suddenly changed? What thoughts are churning in your head? Any memories? Record your observations in your notebook.

6. Depending on the nature of your item, you'll be eating it with a spoon, a fork, or your fingers. Whatever your utensil, eat *the first bite*, allowing yourself to enjoy every sensation—the smells, the crunch in your ear, the texture on your tongue or between your teeth, the distinct taste of salt, sweet, or spice. Is it as you anticipated? Do you have any emotions or past associations? Make notes in your notebook.

7. Repeating the previous step, take one more bite. Then another. Pause between each bite to notice your hunger level and the pleasure you're getting from the food.

8. Continue eating, slowly savoring each bite. Notice how your body is responding to the food and any changes in your pleasure.

9. When it feels like your hunger level is approaching 70% full, stand up and stretch to create more internal space for your treat. Sit back down and continue to eat, noticing if you're getting bored, twitchy, or physically uncomfortable. Does the food still taste as great as the first bites did? If you feel yourself losing enthusiasm, note what percent of the item you've eaten so far. Is it *more* or *less* than you expected to eat before you started this experiment?

10. You have permission to eat every last bite. AND you also have permission to stop eating whenever it no longer pleases you or your stomach.

11. When you've had enough, toss any leftovers in the garbage. Then write about how your body feels and any other thoughts or observations that arise.

12. Postmortem. An hour or two after you complete this exercise notice how your body feels now. Have you had any new realizations?

When you become hyper-focused on the experience of eating a food that has had you under its spell, paying extra attention to each bite will begin to free you from its spell. You will still be able to enjoy it occasionally, but disenchantment has set in. You taste it for for what it is, and now can take it or leave it.

• • • • • REMEMBER THIS • • • • •

- You have more control over how much you eat than you believed.
- Your worst fears, once experienced, are rarely the boogeymen you thought they were.
- The freedom to eat opens the space for the freedom not to eat.

35

Body Break III: Making Amends

Love forgives and keeps no records of wrongs.
—Lailah Gifty Akita

I wasted too many years saying and thinking mean things about certain parts of my body. I was not a kindly caretaker of the only life vessel I'll ever be given. What about you? Have you been mean to your body?

Please take about 15 minutes in this guided meditation to make amends to your body—to apologize to it for ignoring or mistreating it and to give it some love.

Guided Meditation: The Apology and Appreciation Tour. We start with centering breaths, and then, after cultivating a compassionate state of mind, we get into communication with each body part from toe to head, apologizing for any harm we might have done to it and appreciating all it's done for us. The meditation ends with some special affirmations. (Feel free to substitute your own affirmations. In fact, once you get the gist of it, you may want to create and record your own meditation in your phone's voice memo app.)

36

Other People

You've got to start hanging out with friends who fit your future, not your past.

—Internet meme

You likely have friends, family, and coworkers you share meals and stories with. However, because you're making big changes, some people in your life may make reaching your goal more difficult. They are accustomed to the "old you" and may have trouble accepting or believing the new you. They may try your patience, challenge your commitment, and test your ingenuity. Here are two of those tricky situations.

Your Pudgy Pals

If you've been on diets in the past where you became noticeably thinner, or where your friends noticed you were eating different foods or in a different manner, you know that your pudgy pals will be watching your every move. The sad truth is that some may secretly hope you fail. They may even openly subvert your efforts:

"You're going to eat *that*?"

"What crazy diet are you on *now*?"

"How can you possibly lose weight if you can eat whatever you want?"

"You're not finishing your pie? Do you feel OK?"

"No way that plan will work."

"Have one more. It can't hurt."

It's quite possible that *you* may well have been someone's subversive pudgy pal yourself, so you know where this covert hostility comes from: jealousy (because you're succeeding), loss (because misery loves company), and shame (because, if you succeed, it highlights their own failures).

It's doubtful you can change their attitudes or behavior overnight, so you have some choices when you notice these sabotage efforts. 1) Take three deep breaths, politely nod, and keep doing what you were doing. 2) Tell them to shut their trap (not recommended). 3) Find more supportive friends while you're still strengthening your new behaviors.

Understand that your common weight struggles may have been what held certain relationships together. When that commonality dissolves, the friendship may also dissolve. Prepare yourself by exploring other interests and expanding your social circle.

Your Family

If you're the main food preparer for your partner and children, you know how challenging it is to accommodate everyone's food preferences and appetite timing, while staying true to your own program of conscious eating.

I wish I could offer a few easy answers, but every family is unique, and you're going to have to find a way to meet a variety of preferences. An honest conversation about each person's needs around mealtime is a good place to start. These are areas for discussion and probably compromise.

Coordinating schedules. Not everyone can be home to share dinner every night. Work commitments, evening meetings, kids' sports and lessons—all conspire to make it difficult to dine together. Ask everyone involved for input because it's not all on you. What are *their* good ideas? Sometimes you may have to eat before or after others in order to stay true to the Winning Formula.

Appetite timing. Some people are hungriest early in the day (that would be me), and others have appetites that don't arrive until much later (that was my now ex-husband). My ex took my lack of appetite—hence eating so little at dinner—as a personal insult, even though *I* was the one who cooked it. He also couldn't understand how much I enjoyed feasting on leftovers at lunch the next day (he didn't like leftovers).

Food preferences. You like vegetables. They don't. Or vice versa. You're a vegetarian. They're carnivores. Or vice versa. We all have our preferences, and it's futile to argue with personal preferences. I acknowledge it's a huge challenge when you must prepare meals for several others. That's why this is a topic for family discussion. Compromises may be necessary. If you've got some picky eaters, you'll need to be creative in the palate-education game.

Infants and children around the world happily eat all sorts of things we might think are peculiar or inappropriate to introduce until they're much older. If you have small children, Bee Wilson's well-researched book, *First Bite: How We Learn to Eat*, will expand your notions of what's possible. And Virginia Sole-Smith's book, *The Eating Instinct*, will open your mind to the many ways our sometimes strange food preferences develop.

Kids often enjoy taste-testing experiments and ingredient-guessing games, unaware that your goal is to expand the variety of foods they find acceptable. (I played these games with my kids and all three became adventurous eaters and excellent cooks.) With your new experience of how to eat more mindfully and attend to the body's hunger and fullness signals, you can share these skills, thus helping them avoid their own weight problems in the future. You are giving your kids skills that they will appreciate the rest of their lives.

• • • • • REMEMBER THIS • • • • •

- Expect some social friction around your new eating patterns.
- Mental preparation, communication, and compromise will help smooth it.
- Your eating habits set an example for your kids. What kind of example will it be?

37

Social Eating

My doctor told me to stop throwing intimate dinners for four unless there were three other people present.
—Orson Welles

You're on a roll by now. Yay you! You've been very careful to set up your life so that temptations are reduced and mindful behaviors are easier.

But then comes an invitation—a fancy dinner party, a cocktail party, a buffet. Ack!! You want to appear polite, engaged, and appreciative, but worry that maintaining the Winning Formula will be difficult. Maybe the invitation involves people you don't know too well—new neighbors, a potential client, or your boss. Maybe it's from your in-laws or grandmother. What to do?

Mental preparation is essential, which means first considering your purpose in attending and the outcome you desire as a result of being there. Here's one trick I use to set myself up for success in a variety of situations that might be challenging: I ask myself how my *future self—the self I'll be tomorrow or some time down the road*—would like to see the situation played out as I look back. And then I imagine how I could make that happen. Each scenario below requires a slightly different approach, but they all start with purpose and intention.

The Dinner Party

What is your purpose in attending? Is it to get into or stay in your host's good graces? Do you hope to know the other guests better, to discover common ground? You don't have to clean your plate with enthusiasm to prove you're a worthy guest. If you're shy and would rather not attract attention to yourself, focus on the other person(s). When you ask open-ended questions and listen carefully to what they say, the focus is off you (and what you are *not* eating), and it makes them feel special. Win-win.

What eating behaviors seem most risky in this situation? Will the second glass of wine lower your resistance to accepting seconds? If you leave some food on your plate, do you fear your host's feelings will be hurt? Will you lose track of your hunger levels if the meal goes on and on?

How will you be polite? If you're pressed to eat more, how will you shut down your inner **Martyr**? What phrases will you use to explain your behaviors? The people most likely to press you are family members and good friends "who knew you when" you were a bottomless pit. *You do not need to apologize for eating less. "True thins" never do.* No explanation is needed beyond, "It was delicious. I have no space left for another bite."

Practice your "out." Whatever statement you decide to use as your out, repeat it to yourself several times with conviction. You may never need it, but repetition will serve to strengthen your inner resolve.

The Cocktail or Networking Party

Prepare yourself ahead of time as above by setting your intention for the event. If alcoholic beverages are involved, understand how your inhibitions are reduced after one drink (after two?). It's best to stay away from the bar and shake your head no when the tasty hors d'oeuvres come around for the second or third time. Remember, you're there to connect with other people.

After I donned my scientific observer hat, I discovered that I'd been using my wine glass and snack plate as introvert crutches. Whenever I felt uncomfortable, I would take a sip from my glass or wave it around, or refill my plate and say something obvious about the appetizer, the food version of "How 'bout them Yankees!" This was a poor strategy for connecting more deeply with other guests.

Instead, I decided to spend the first 30 to 60 minutes empty-handed—no glass, no plate—so I could focus my full attention on the person or people I was talking to. When I stopped worrying about making a good impression and instead tried to get to know what got the person up in the morning, we both had a more rewarding interaction. [Insider tip #1: Other people worry about making a good impression on *you*, so forget about yourself and focus on them. They will think you're brilliant.]

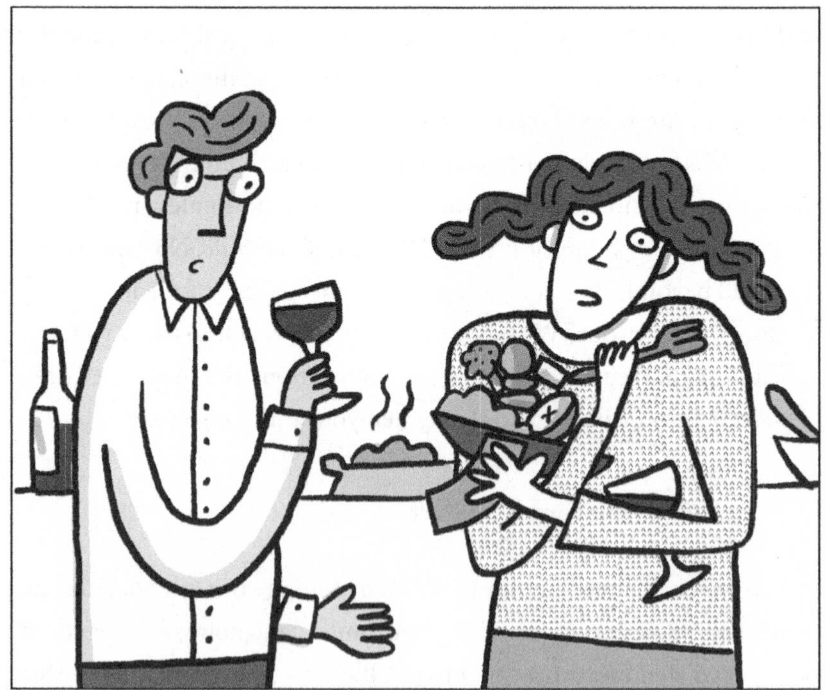

The Bottomless Buffet or Perfect Potluck

In this instance, your intention might have an additional twist—you want to taste new foods or enjoy old favorites you'd never make for yourself. The buffet is full of Teasers. It brings out our FOMO (Fear of Missing Out)—we want to try *everything*.

Envision the serving table, laden with all sorts of foods—so many dishes, so little stomach space! Some foods will be old standbys—on the appetizer end: raw veggies with hummus dip, crackers, cheeses, and cold cuts—on the dessert end: brownies, lemon bars, and chocolate chip cookies. But wait! You may also find dishes you don't recognize or haven't enjoyed in a long time.

What will be your strategy? Will you go for old favorites or new tastes? Eat dessert first? Only salads? Just one bite of each and every dish? How will you deal with a big helping of something that looked delicious on the platter but turns out to be *meh?* How will you handle your concern that everyone's watching and thinking, "No wonder she weighs so much! Look at the pile on her plate!" [Insider tip #2: Most people are thinking about what's on their own plates, not what's on yours.]

The line forms to the left. Already you can smell the delicious temptations ahead. Do not charge into the line, napkin under your chin. Wait until it has thinned, because you are going to take your own sweet time choosing what to put on your plate.

Before you pick up a plate, walk the entire length of the table and scope out the scene. What is familiar and what's new? What intrigues you? If you'd envisioned eating dessert first or only eating salads, does the dessert or salad plan still look viable?

Now get your plate and go down the line again, serving yourself *small amounts* of what you mentally chose. It's OK to choose nothing but desserts. If a food turns out to be super delicious, you can always go back for more. And if it's disappointing, don't feel bad about leaving it on the plate or slipping it into the trash. A "true thin" would do that without a second thought.

Find a seat and do your best to set aside expectations from prior experience with each food sample. Focus on the taste and texture in your mouth at this moment. Can you discern the ingredients? What makes it pleasing or not so pleasing? Is it worth eating or should you move on to the next sample?

As soon as you feel sufficiently fed, toss your plate and *step away from the food trough.*

Prompt: Do a postmortem. Whatever kind of party it was, when you get back home, review the event and make notes in your notebook. Acknowledge yourself for every little thing that went well. If you were less than pleased with some of your behaviors, how might you do better next time?

• • • • • REMEMBER THIS • • • • •

- Prepare by setting a clear intention and strategy for the event ahead of time.
- Ask yourself, "WWTTD?"—What Would a "True Thin" Do?
- Any setback is a powerful opportunity for learning.

PART SIX

Practice and Persist

Learning any new skill takes practice, patience, and persistence. You will have setbacks from time to time. How do you keep going when you feel discouraged?

And what will you do after (when) you arrive at your goal? It's time to look at the bigger picture.

38

Nutrition and Exercise Do Matter

All right. It's come to this. We need to talk about the quality of the food you eat and what you're doing to burn up those calories you've consumed.

Just because I've made no mention so far about what you should or shouldn't eat, or about exercise as a component of a healthy lifestyle, doesn't mean they don't matter. Far from it. I didn't go back to school for a graduate degree in public health for nothing. I believe passionately in the importance of both nutrition and exercise.

The primary goal of this book is to help you flip your fat-mindset 180°—to help you establish a sane, truthful, present-moment relationship with food and to let go of those attitudes, beliefs, and behaviors that keep you stuck in the yo-yo syndrome. Once you've given yourself permission to slowly savor a variety of previously "forbidden" foods, pigged out on all the donuts, and discovered why you find French fries so irresistible (and really, braving these delicious dragons *mano a mano* must come first), it's time to talk about your long-term health.

Food First

In this life practice of being *a mindful eater*, no foods are off limits unless your doctor tells you so. However, not all food is created equal. Our poor food choices are worse killers than smoking or alcohol. We are overfed and undernourished.

We used to be hunter/gatherers. Now our foods are hunting us. As we've gotten busier and lazier about cooking for ourselves, we're assaulted on all sides by unhealthy quick and easy options. Processed oils and fats lurk everywhere, even in instant noodles. We're consuming 30% more sugar than we did in the 1970s—especially in drinks: sodas, fruit juices, specialty coffee and tea concoctions, alcoholic beverages. Drinks can account for several hundred thoughtless calories a day.

It's time to choose foods that are beneficial to your remarkable body. When Michael Pollan, author of the bestseller *In Defense of Food*, says, "Eat food. Not too much. Mostly plants." he means *real* foods that don't come in packages or bags or cans or large plastic bottles—real foods that are found on the outer aisles of your supermarket, not on the Teaser displays near the check stand.

It's true that nutritious food costs more initially and will require more time and effort to put on the table. However, flip your thinking. Healthy food is not an expense, it's an *investment* that pays off by improving your health and reducing future medical costs.

My favorite books on healthful eating aren't diet books. They're cookbooks that focus on preparing vegetables in interesting ways or ones that introduce my palate to the new flavors of different ethnic cuisines. My commitment to healthy eating always gets stronger when I read about the food industry and how it operates to cut costs and ensnare consumers (see readings for chapter 2).

In his books, Michael Pollan focuses on the nature of our current food supply, how to determine what's good for both us and the planet, and how to improve our eating habits in a way that suits our own particular preferences. Three of my favorite of Pollan's food rules, from another of his books, *Food Rules*:

Don't eat anything your great-grandmother wouldn't recognize as food.

Avoid foods you see advertised on television.

If it came from a plant, eat it; if it was made in a plant, don't.

The bottom line: Do your best to avoid foods low in nutrients and fiber and/or high in sugars, fats, flavorings, and preservatives. More than half of the calorie intake in the United States comes from processed foods, including sweetened breakfast cereals, granola bars, fruit yogurt, candy, chicken nuggets, hot dogs, instant noodles and similar mixes, soft drinks, and those liquid desserts masquerading as fancy coffee drinks at Starbucks. Profit margins are highest in the junk food category because food manufacturers use cheap ingredients that have a long shelf life. The per calorie cost to the consumer may be cheaper, but it comes at the expense of your health.

Practice: Learn to cook *real* food, if you don't already know how. There are YouTube videos that will teach you everything from knife skills (the best way to chop an onion or cut up a chicken) to making your own salad dressing, cooking up a mess of chili, or whipping up a soufflé. A million recipes await you for free on the internet. You could even crack an old school cookbook.

Move It!

The challenge with starting a new exercise regime is just that—*starting*. I have fallen off the exercise wagon several times in my life. Each time, my resistance to starting over was hard to overcome because I knew how out of shape I'd gotten. To restart would prove my weakness, not just physically but willpower-wise. The only way to get around my mental block was by setting my standards for accomplishment laughably low. The slightest effort earned me a check mark on the calendar. I walked to the corner ☑. I did one pushup ☑. I danced "R-E-S-P-E-C-T" with Aretha Franklin ☑.

The first few times, that was all I did. Of course, once I'd made the effort to put on the shoes, get down on the floor, or turn up the music, it became easier to keep going. One pushup became two, which became five, and so forth. There were days when time constraints or low motivation held me back, but I could still manage to keep up my winning streak by doing *one* pushup.

The key to creating a successful exercise program is managing what's going on in your mind, just like in the rest of your life. When your mind thinks something is going to be hard or unpleasant, it balks. It throws up a dozen creative excuses and a hundred stories about why it's a stupid idea, that you don't really feel like it, and that now is not really a good time.

How do you shut down your resistance before it shuts *you* down? You give yourself a nonnegotiable countdown: *5-4-3-2-1 Go!* That's how. I learned this from Mel Robbins, whose book, *The 5-Second Rule,* is all about acting immediately on your intention *before* you fall for one of your oh-so-excellent excuses. You've set your timer to remind yourself to take a walk in one hour. The timer dings, your resistance remembers a phone call that must be made *now.* Nope, you made a commitment to yourself, so before your mind can take over, you count down: *5-4-3-2-1 Go!* You put on your walking shoes and step out the door.

Walking requires only that you have comfortable shoes and weather-appropriate outer wear. If you walk alone, it's a great time to use all your senses to appreciate where you are. You can also plug in your headset and boost your spirit listening to happy music or learn something from a podcast. If you have trouble keeping commitments with yourself (and many people do, including yours truly), enroll a friend to join you. In my running days, I needed a partner to be accountable to, or I wouldn't do it.

I'm also a believer in the wonders of yoga, not just to increase your strength and flexibility, but also to reduce stress, help you connect you with your body, and bring you into the present moment. I prefer live classes, however you'll find many at every level of competence on YouTube and inexpensive mobile phone apps. And of course, there's always dancing—in your home to '80s disco music, online for a salsa or hip-hop class, or live, where the energy of the group feeds you and you can ask the teacher for help. What's important is that you MOVE.

Exercise is a positive habit that must be established and maintained, just like any other habit. The books on habit change by James Clear, Gretchen Rubin, and Charles Duhigg are terrific on the subject of creating a solid exercise habit (see resources for Chapter 29 in Appendix C).

Practice: Daily Exercise. Commit to physical movement every day. Get yourself a wall calendar and some gold stars or happy face stickers and give yourself one each day you move, even if it's one pushup. Seeing 30 gold stars on the calendar will motivate you to keep going.

REMEMBER THIS

- Our poor food choices are worse killers than smoking or alcohol.
- Nutritious food is an investment in better health and reduced medical costs.
- The hardest step in any exercise program is the first one.

39

Plateaus and the Plague of Perfectionism

Don't let the perfect be the enemy of the good.
—Italian aphorism

You've made it thus far on your journey toward freedom from weight obsession. You've shed some weight at a slow and steady pace. You're feeling much more in control of your eating.

Then... uh-oh! At some point, your progress levels off. Your waistband is exactly as tight today as it was last week. The needle on your scales seems stuck (though I hope you're no longer relying on it—see chapter 5). Memories of every other time you hit this plateau begin to infect your thoughts. It feels depressingly like the last time you got here. *Déjà vu* all over again. You consider a run to the store for a gallon of Ben and Jerry's.

Nooooo! That is your fat machinery kicking in, unwilling to give up its grip on your mind. I don't want to get all technical on you, because this is not that kind of book, but let me remind you of what's called "set-point theory." It states that your body has a natural weight, which it seeks to maintain. Once your weight dips below (or above) its set point, especially if it happens quickly, your metabolism adjusts in an attempt to restore that particular weight. Hence the plateau. This is one reason that I advocate sneaking up on your set point by losing weight very gradually over time. That way, the body doesn't slow down your metabolism to conserve calories because it thinks it's starving.

Is this the end of the line? It is possible that your body is genetically designed to hang out at this predetermined destination regardless of what you do. You have *arrived*, even if you aren't yet ready to accept it. My hope is that you've become more appreciative of the body you have at every step on this journey, at each weight point. *It is what it is*, and you're lucky to have it.

It is also possible that you've just hit a rest stop—a flat place on your mountain hike where you put down your pack, eat your apple, drink some water, and take in the view.

Either way, do not give up eating consciously just because your weight seems to be stuck. As you survey the view below, acknowledge yourself for how far you've come on this journey, how much you've learned about yourself, how much more you enjoy your food, and how much energy you've already freed for other areas of your life.

Is The Perfectionist one of your inner pirates? Join the crowd. We look out at our peers, or at least at the images they project (which probably hide their own insecurities), and by comparison, we do not measure up. We keep thinking *if only* I were [nicer, smarter, prettier, hipper, stronger, funnier, thinner, like so-and-so], *then* I'd be happy, or the cool guy would pick me, or I'd get the best job, or...

Let's be realistic here. None of us are perfect. The skinny model is moody and humorless. The hip professor isn't on speaking terms with anyone in his family. The comedian is very funny, but damn, she's even more insecure than you. Behind your perfect idol is someone who would kill for your happy marriage or your rewarding career. Whose standards are you trying to meet, anyway? (See chapter 14.)

Becoming a healthy eater is a life practice, not an end point. The reason many activities we do (yoga, sports, playing an instrument, meditation, doctoring or lawyering) are called *practices* is because there is no perfect endpoint. We do them for the doing. As beautifully as Yo-Yo Ma plays the cello, he never thinks he's arrived at perfection; he keeps on practicing every day.

✏📖 **Prompt: Plateau Report.** Write about your experience of this plateau. How does it feel compared to previous plateaus? What have you learned about your relationship to food and eating so far? Has it changed? How are you and your body getting along these days—are you on better terms? What beliefs and old stories have you brought into the light? Have you dropped any of those? **Go back through your notebook and create a list of victories big and small, and then acknowledge yourself. Yay, you!**

Is It Time to Give Yourself Some Loving Kindness?

For a kinder lighter relationship to yourself over the long haul, I believe a regular meditation practice can't be beat. For meditation skeptics, ABC newsman Dan Harris's bestseller, *10% Happier*, describes his road to recovery from his inner trash-talker, using meditation. His popular weekly podcast and meditation app, *Ten Percent Happier*, will introduce you to a variety of perspectives on the practice. For a beginning meditator it really helps to be guided by an experienced teacher, and this app has some of the best.

Doing a short guided meditation every day helps you recognize that you are not your thoughts, feelings or stories. You're more able to watch them come and go without getting caught up in them, which makes it easier to roll with life's punches. As your inner judge recedes, you develop more compassion towards yourself and others. Win-win-win.

But what about the stress you're feeling right now? You've had a hard day/week/year/life. You'd like a little treat… but an ice cream sundae or a pile of French fries seems counterproductive. Any time is a good time to try one of these:

- **Power nap.** Set a timer for 20 minutes and stretch out on the couch or even better, if you can—on the floor with your lower legs raised on a bolster or foot stool (in yoga class, we call that *savasana*). This is short enough for a mental reboot, but not so long that you awaken in a fog. Close your eyes and take a few deep breaths. Let your neck and shoulders loosen and drop, because they're tight, right? Allow your mind to drift. The intention is not to sleep, but to reboot your brain, clearing away the day's accumulation of mental sludge.

- **Have a drink (of water).** Alcoholic beverages can make you feel better briefly, but millions of American women are drinking more than ever before. Habitual happy hours do not foster losing weight.
- **Move!** [I know, I'm repeating myself, but I mean it.] Put your headset on, tune your phone to whatever music makes you want to dance, and spend 10 minutes getting into your body. Step outside, even if it's raining—*especially* if it's raining. Use Body Break II in chapter 25 to rev up your ch'i.
- **Call someone.** Think of a person you enjoy but haven't spoken with in some time—former coworkers, friends, cousins. Make a list of them, and then pick up the phone and call the first person on the list to say hi. This is not a call for help; you just want to connect and hear what they're up to. This call is not about you; it's about connection.
- **Pamper yourself.** Throw in the towel for the day and do something completely frivolous. Take a bubble bath, get a pedicure or massage, buy some fresh flowers and make a beautiful arrangement, start a jigsaw puzzle, read a trashy novel, go to a movie matinee.

Prompt: Write your own list of self-care ideas—short breaks or bigger treats. Slot them into your life as often as you can.

Alrighty then, plateau break over. Lurch back onto your feet and carry on. We'll address more serious setbacks in the next chapter.

REMEMBER THIS

- Successful living is a daily practice.
- You'll never be perfect, so enjoy the ride.

40

Recovering From Setbacks

Failures are painful, but once I stop beating myself up, they always teach me something valuable.

—Janette B., Thin Within participant

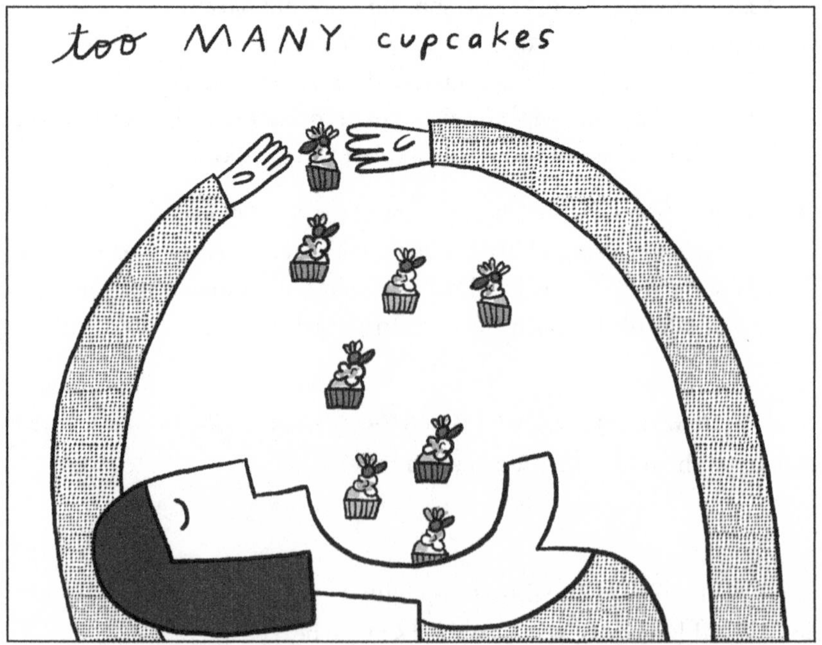

Over the next few months, you *will* experience setbacks—moments when you're sure you're headed for yet another embarrassing failure. You get on the scales and the readout hasn't budged. You eat all the cupcakes.

Setbacks happen. You've struggled with your weight for years, so don't expect to resolve your issues in a few weeks. Be like the tortoise:

slow and steady wins the race. Your positive habits compound over time to bring lasting results.

Remember, the process is often three steps forward and one step back, over and over and over. Instead of getting so discouraged you quit, do some troubleshooting. Here are some places to explore:

- **Don't like what the scales said? Toss them.** Then pay closer attention to your hunger signals and stop eating a little sooner. Instead, rely on the fit of your clothes. Looser, tighter, or the same?

- **You haven't set up your life so it works for you.** You put yourself in the way of temptations that are hard to resist—**The Willing Victim.** For example, you still keep your pantry stocked with snack foods and soft drinks. You find excuses to walk by the fancy bakery with the tantalizing fragrances wafting onto the street. You hang out by the buffet table at a party. You refuse to set aside time to enjoy your meals in relative peace.

- **You forgot you are the *chooser*, not the victim. Choice is your super power.** To do or not to do? To eat or not to eat? This means you must be alert to the stories (lies) you tell yourself. If you tell yourself "I can't eat just one __," or "I can't resist __," recognize that these are lies. What you're really saying is "I *won't* eat only one __," and "I *refuse* to resist __." Because you absolutely have it in your power to choose.

  The empowering truth is this: "**I *can* eat just one, and I'm *choosing* to eat five.**" "I *can* resist chocolate, and right now I'm *choosing* to eat this truffle." Telling the truth in this manner puts you in the driver's seat; you're no longer the victim of your "uncontrollable" whims. Eating more healthfully is not a *sacrifice*, it is the route to a goal that *you chose*. And must continue to choose, moment by moment.

- **You forgot that your weight is a *project*, not a *problem*.** Like all projects, it consists of many elements. Break it down into manageable chunks—action steps you can succeed at. Here are some sample action steps you could take on, a *week at a time*:

- Get back in touch with your body's hunger and fullness signals by charting them again (SuperTool #1).
- Focus on really tasting your food, especially after the first flavor flush is gone. Rate everything (1 to 10) and consider leaving anything that rates 5 or below (SuperTool #4).
- Eat more fruits and vegetables.
- Explore. Try new ethnic cuisines. Try eating some foods you disliked as a kid. Experiment with herbs, spices and condiments.
- Eliminate snacks and after-dinner eating. Are you succumbing to too many Teasers (SuperTool #5)?
- Cut back or eliminate alcoholic beverages. They weaken your resolve.
- Beautify your table as if you were entertaining someone special (because you *are* special). Sit at it and feel special every time you eat.
- Create artful arrangements of the food on your plate, as if you were a chef at a fancy restaurant or a floral designer.
- Say a prayer of gratitude for each thing on your plate, and for all who got it there.

➤ **In case of catastrophe, look for the lessons.** Separate the facts of what happened from your excuses and judgments. Take an alternative view: at least you didn't eat *two* platefuls of brownies. As the saying goes, "Never let a crisis go to waste." Were you responding to an emotional trigger? What happened to create this situation? What would have been a better move on your part? When this mood or situation happens again—it will—how will you deal more effectively? Remember the rocket ship (chapter 33). Get back on course.

➤ **You've forgotten to pay loving attention to your body.** It's the only one you've got, and many people are counting on you sticking around in it—in good health. Does it need to stretch? Does it need more sleep?

Is it thirsty? Does it need to get out in nature? Would it prefer more nutritious foods? Are you clothing it in attractive garments that flatter you? Find an enjoyable movement practice and do it.

➤ **You're resisting the Winning Formula (SuperTool #3).** The purpose of the Winning Formula is to create an environment most likely to give you the results *you say you want*. So why are you resisting? Here are some favorite excuses:

- *I'm just too busy*. Fine. Whatever. I call bullshit. Getting rid of your weight worries once and for all was *your* idea.
- *I'm a rebel and don't like discipline*. This attitude hurts you, not me. Reframe the practice as a devotional—to yourself—for your own benefit and for the benefit of those who love and depend on you. You're building better eating habits for a lifetime.
- *I'm pissed off that I can't eat as much as I want*. (Your fuel gauge hit 70% but your eyes or emotions still covet more). To counteract this, slooow down and focus on savoring the food that is currently in your mouth.
- *I don't like paying so much attention to eating*. It's boring. It feels self-indulgent. It brings up uncomfortable thoughts. Good. Welcome those thoughts to the table where you can look them in the eye and tell them to get lost; you deserve this time to nourish yourself.

➤ **You fell back in with your old dieting crowd** who tell you you're nuts—you really must try this new diet that's all the rage. Swear off those folks until you find solid footing (chapter 36).

➤ **You forgot to notice and acknowledge how far you've come.** Fight your negativity bias and **celebrate every win**. Write them down in your notebook on a special page you can turn to when you need encouragement or create a Wins Jar (a container that's your piggy bank for depositing slips of paper noting each tiny victory). Listen to or repeat your affirmations every day. They may be stories, but they're supportive stories, not saboteurs. Don't forget you can always create fresh affirmations for new issues and special occasions.

- **You stopped using your notebook.** It's a great dumping ground for toxic thoughts that you don't want polluting your mind. Keep track of your progress and brilliant insights. Give yourself gold stars or smiley face stickers. Try your hand at writing food poetry (an ode to jelly donuts), food porn (five ways to use butter) or food rants (hate mail to kale).
- **You're intimidated by the idea of eating like this *forever*.** Eating mindfully should become more pleasurable than your old ways. However, if the idea of maintaining this practice for life freaks you out, do it one day at a time, one meal at a time. (Over and over.)
- **Final pitfall—you reach your weight goal and realize you're still not content:** Prince Charming didn't show up, you didn't get the job of your dreams, you're still unsatisfied with your life. Guess what: you're human. Humans actually need ~~problems~~, I mean *projects*, to feel alive, to give us something to do.

• • • • • REMEMBER THIS • • • • •

- You're meant for a bigger game. That's what's next...

41

Life Is a Game

Life is a game. In order to have a game, something
has to be more important than something else.
If ***what already is****, is more important than* ***what isn't****,*
the game is over. So, life is a game in which
what isn't is more important than what is.
Let the good times roll.
—Werner Erhard

We're almost at the end of our time together on these pages. How are you doing?

✏📖 **Prompt: Fill out the "After" questionnaire.** Copy the questions from Appendix A into your notebook, or download a blank version in Word from my website. Then compare it to your "Before" answers to note what has changed.

Think of your weight project as a game. At the moment, it's pretty engaging. Getting to your goal (*what isn't, yet*) is more important than your present body (*what is, now*). Maybe you have been a yo-yo dieter and you've played this game many times. Except I hope this time, it *is* different—you reach your goal once and for all—your fat-mindset is gone, and the extra pounds are slipping off. Game over. The victory feels fantastic. For at least a week, maybe even a month.

Then the thrill wears off and life continues as before. As the Zen master said, when asked what happens after you reach enlightenment, "Chop wood, carry water."

If you think reaching your weight goal is a challenge, try getting to the moon! That was astronaut Buzz Aldrin's life goal, and in 1969 he stepped onto the lunar surface. However, after achieving such a literal high, he'd neglected to think about life when he came down. All the time and energy he had previously occupied with intensive training had no place to go. Without a new vision, he sank into depression and alcoholism.

I'm not saying that's where you're headed, but if your weight ~~problem~~ project has taken a big chunk of your focus and you complete it, a large hole opens up in front of you, sometimes revealing how the problem let you off the hook for other issues needing attention. I love how James Baldwin expressed this dilemma: "Nothing is more desirable than to be released from an affliction, but nothing is more frightening than to be divested of a crutch."

Nature abhors a vacuum. So do human beings. Empty space makes us anxious; in our discomfort, we want to fill it. The easiest solution is to revert to your old ways—overeating and weight obsessing. Again.

That's how I responded to Edward's death. The time and energy I'd focused on the demands of his illness for two years were no longer needed. Overnight, a giant hole appeared where my husband and his care had been. I was frightened by the empty space and the uncertainty about what might come next.

In *Transitions*, the classic book about coping with major life changes, William Bridges suggests that the end of something big is not really the *end*, it's the *beginning* of what's to come. Something must end in order to create space for something new. That makes some sense. Unfortunately, before we discover what's to come, we must dwell for an uncomfortable period in the *emptiness of not knowing, of uncertainty.*

We human beings do not like *not knowing*. We do not like uncertainty.

Tibetan Buddhists call this empty space the *bardo*—an intermediate, transitional, or liminal state between death and rebirth. As the monk Yongey Mingyur Rinpoche says, "I am in the bardo of becoming right now, between the death of the old me and the birth of whatever comes next. Becoming and becoming, always in the bardo of the unknown, the uncertain, the transient."

The *bardo* is also a metaphorical way to describe times when our usual way of life becomes suspended, like during a period of intense preoccupation with a problem—for example having to shelter in place because of a pandemic. The challenge becomes this: will we use this *bardo* for spiritual progress or will we fall back on our less skillful impulses?

Being at your goal is not the end in itself; it's a *means to an end*. You're creating the space for the real game—living your *why*. So, get out your notebook and prepare to spend a little time envisioning your future. However, we're going to do it from the opposite end—from your 88th birthday *looking back* at your life.

I offer you three thought experiments and invite you to write your responses to them:

✎📖 **Prompt #1: *Imagine you just celebrated your 88th birthday.*** *Friends and family are toasting you with champagne. The cake is totally covered with candles. Can you see it? OK, good. Now* ***imagine that you still haven't resolved your weight problem****—your size hasn't changed, and you still feel like food is the enemy. What specifically did you do to maintain that same old weight problem? As you look back over those decades, what were the consequences of* ***never*** *resolving your weight problem? Did it impact other areas of your life? In what ways?*

✎📖 **Prompt #2: Rewind the tape *back to the candle-laden cake and your 88th birthday. This time imagine that you resolved your weight project*** *long, long ago—within a year of completing this process. Congratulations! What specifically did you do to dismantle that old weight problem? As you look back over those decades, what were the consequences of resolving your weight problem? Did it impact other areas of your life? In what ways?*

✏📖 **Prompt #3: Uh-Oh.** Shortly after your 88th birthday celebration, you get backed over by a Budweiser beer truck. No problem—you knew you wouldn't live forever, so you planned ahead and ordered your gravestone, complete with an epitaph you crafted yourself. It says: "Here lies _____. She lost 57 pounds in 2021 and stayed slim the rest of her life." Well, yay you. But is that all you want for yourself?

Do you not have bigger fish to fry in this lifetime? If your epitaph had space to describe a particular contribution or purpose that would make you proud, what might it say? "Here lies _____. He served 10,000 Meals-on-Wheels."

If you're drawing a blank on your epitaph, not to worry… in the bardo, you have all the time you need to ponder this important question and set the stage to make it happen.

• • • • • REMEMBER THIS • • • • •

- Being at your goal is a means to an end, not the end itself.
- The bardo is an invitation to curiosity and discovery.
- What new game will you create?

42

So Where's the Cherry Pie?

To change one's life, start immediately. Do it flamboyantly.
—William James

You now have my complete toolbox, and you're on your way. Maybe you've already arrived at your goal—you've let go of counterproductive habits, developed a more conscious and choosy palate, made peace with food and your body, and you may now find yourself at your ideal weight. The *Cherry Pie* ***Paradox*** is that you can have your pie and eat it *without guilt*.

And yet the angels have not yet sung, you're not yet in shape for the Boston Marathon, and dirty dishes await you in the sink. As I said at the outset, your weight "problem" was never the real problem. It was an obstacle on the path to getting on with the real work of your life. You turned this tired *problem* into a *project* with action steps that would help you meet it head on and blast through it.

What lies ahead is the *real cherry pie*: the freedom to express your unique contribution to your loved ones and the rest of the world. You may have no idea what that might look like, or you may have caught a glimpse of it when you looked back from your 88th birthday or when you remember your *why*.

To be sure, as soon as you identify a new goal, obstacles will arise in the path. That's just what happens when you set a goal. The biggest obstacle is usually the trash-talker in your head, and you now have some tools to deal with that saboteur. (Hint: start by turning the *problem* into a *project* with action steps, then engage your curiosity and inner scientist, taking any missteps as learning opportunities.)

If you're still in the throes of your weight wars, remember, it took *years* for you to solidify this problem. Give yourself time to undo the damage, *and* don't slack off. I know you can do it because thousands of Thin Within participants did it before you. Just last year a woman tracked me down on Facebook, despite four decades and my name change. She now runs The Red Tractor Farm, an inn on the Greek island of Kea.

> *Dear Joy,*
>
> *Many years ago, I had the transformative experience of attending a Thin Within course that you taught in Palo Alto, California. I hadn't thought much about that seminar for a long time, even though it obviously changed my entire relationship with food, and made me into a lifelong mindful eater.*
>
> *I've begun writing* The Red Tractor Farm Book, *a compilation of recipes, thoughts, and tips from what we have learned running our inn. As I write about food, I realize that something must be shared about* ***how*** *we eat, not just* ***what*** *we eat; hence my sudden remembrance of you and the amazing work you did in the founding of Thin Within.*
>
> *So, this is a thank-you note from someone on whose life you effected profound, positive change nearly forty years ago.*
>
> *Best wishes,*
>
> *Marcie Mayer*

Keep Going!

In this, our final guided meditation, you'll connect again with your healthy beloved body. It concludes with affirmations.

Guided Meditation: My Healthy Beloved Body.

My wish for you is that this practice becomes such an invisible part of your life, you can't even remember how you used to fuss about your weight. I hope that you find ways to extend the reach of the awareness skills you've cultivated here into many other arenas.

Dip back into this book on a regular basis. Reread a couple of chapters and repeat a writing prompt, taste test or guided meditation. Work your way through it with a few friends (positivity partners).With each visit, you'll bring a wiser self. You'll make new connections and deepen your appreciation for the life-changing power of this work.

I don't exaggerate; following this process is life-changing.

Revise and expand your affirmations. Create your own eating experiences or rituals. Think about other ways you can lighten up in your relationship to food—write about it, as I did in my cottage cheese rant (chapter 27); play with it, as I describe in the epilogue; or sing about it, as former Thin Within participant Alva did (chapter 25).

Even though I only had twelve pounds to shed by the time I finally gave up dieting and started Thin Within, it took many months of practicing the tools to work through the garbage in my head. One day at a party I was offered a piece of fudge cake, and only later did I notice that I accepted it because I was hungry; it never crossed my mind to ask myself that automatic old question: "how fattening is this?" It was then I realized my "weight problem" had evaporated.

The journey reminds me of *The Very Hungry Caterpillar* by Eric Carle, a favorite board book when my kids were little. To summarize: the caterpillar hatches from an egg, gets hungry, and begins eating. First, he eats a hole in an apple. "But he was STILL hungry!" So, he eats a hole in each of two pears. "But he was STILL hungry!" He eats a hole in each of three plums. After each "meal," the line is, "But he was STILL hungry!" Every day for a week, he eats and grows bigger and bigger. On his final day as a caterpillar, he eats so much junk food that he gets a stomachache. Soon after, he wraps himself in a cocoon.

And you know what happens next.

Isn't that how too many of us live our lives—STILL hungry for something, but not knowing what? As we metaphorically consume life experiences and hit that dark-night-of-the-soul stomachache, we remain hopeful we *will* be reborn, more amazing and beautiful than we could have ever imagined. May it be so for you.

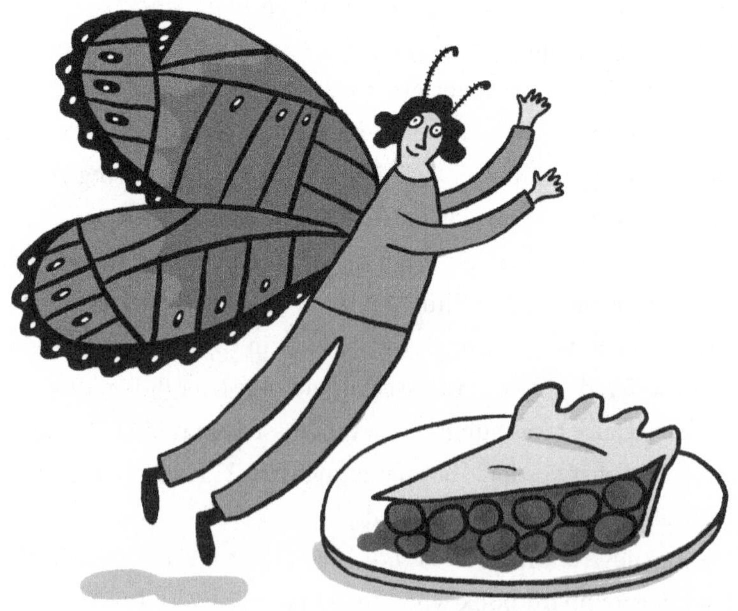

So *namaste* and thank you, my friend. I am grateful you've given me the opportunity to share this transformative practice with you. Keep being curious. Keep going. And keep in touch.

• • • • • REMEMBER THIS • • • • •

- Stay curious.
- Be kind to yourself.
- Practice. Practice. Practice!
- *You can do this!*

Epilogue

Time to Play

In late spring, the PTA at the kids' elementary school always held a fund-raising carnival. In years past, I'd run the popcorn booth, the bean bag toss, the pie competition. My job in 1979 was to oversee the popular hot dog booth, which always attracted a swarm of hungry kids eager to spend their pink tickets. By the end of the afternoon, we'd run out of hot dogs but still had extra buns, ketchup, pickle relish, mustard, and popcorn. The sandwich booth next to mine had a surfeit of grape jelly and Skippy peanut butter. The trash barrels were rolled out to collect all the leftovers.

As anyone obsessed with food knows, it's a sin to throw away perfectly good food. At least, that was what I once believed.

"I'll take it home," I told the carnival chairperson.

"What will you do with it?" she asked with one raised eyebrow. "It's crap. People have had their fingers in it; it's been sitting out all day."

I knew it was crap, and I didn't yet have a plan, but something would come to me. I still loved the challenge of improvising with leftovers—the culinary version of making a silk purse out of a sow's ear.

Once I got home, I placed the array of jars, bottles, and bags of crap on the kitchen counter and contemplated what to do next. In its post-carnival state, the food was probably not safe to eat. Then I had an idea so exhilarating it took my breath away.

"Heather! Ethan! Come down to the kitchen right now, and bring your painting aprons."

Mystified, they traipsed into the kitchen. I tied on their aprons.

"We're going to play with our food," I announced.

They stared at me. Playing with food? What?

Playing with food had always been *verboten,* going way back in our family history. Food was for eating. Period. My mom believed it was immoral to play with something so precious when children around the world went hungry. At the end of a meal, if we still had food on our plates, our only option was to sit quietly with our hands in our lap waiting to be excused from the table. But now Mom wasn't watching.

My kitchen was a cook's dream. It featured a narrow center island with an inlaid cutting board edged with Mexican tiles. On the far side were three stools, where we sat to eat most of our meals. The other side was my "chef's station" from whence I chopped, sautéed, and slung hash in the kids' direction.

I plunked Heather and Ethan on the stools. From my side, I opened all the containers and bags and heaped their contents onto the counter. I augmented our materials with some stale Cheerios and too-dry raisins from one cabinet, and some droopy celery and broccoli stalks from the fridge.

I distributed butter knives and spoons. "OK, kids. You can spread this stuff anywhere you want on the countertop. You can make roads through it; you can make little mountains or gardens or forests. Have at it!"

They were so certain I was putting them on that they just sat there, confused.

"I mean it! Here, I'll start."

I spread a thick layer of peanut butter down the center of the counter and added a ribbon of grape jelly. "This is a brook," I said. I squished a hot dog bun next to the brook. "Here's a stone wall."

The dam of reluctance broke, and they dove in. For the next hour, the three of us sculpted our gloppy village with glee. Ethan pushed one of his Matchbox cars down his sticky road, and Heather placed several of her Fisher-Price people in the broccoli-tree forest.

For them, it was the Best Game Ever—flouting the rules with the rule-maker herself. For me, it represented my hard-won freedom from food obsession. I wish I'd had a tiny flag to plant like a conquering hero atop the pickle relish hill.

Under normal circumstances, I'd *hate* cleaning up such a stupendous mess, but not this time. For the kids' amusement, I pretended to be a bulldozer, complete with sound effects, as I scraped section after section of our construction into the garbage can. It exceeded by far the amount of food I'd ever trashed in one swoop, and I did it without a pang of guilt. As I restored the countertop to its usual state, I reflected on how far I'd come in the past few years.

I hadn't worried about the food I had (or hadn't) eaten and what I weighed (or didn't weigh) for months! The last vestiges of an enormous emotional burden that had nearly killed me a few years earlier were gone, *and I hadn't even noticed.* My fat-mindset had evaporated, never again to rear her conniving head, and food regained its rightful place as a nurturing pleasure instead of the enemy waiting to ambush me and suck me into its greedy grasp.

And that, my friends, is what a transformation looks like.

How will *you* celebrate?

Appendices

APPENDIX A:
Questionnaires, Forms and Winning Formula

You can easily draw the food diary forms and many of the charts yourself in your notebook. However, they're all available as blanks for you to download from the private folder on my website: joyoverstreet.com/pie. The two questionnaires online are in Word document format so you will have all the space you need to properly fill them out. All the materials are organized by chapter.

Introduction: The "Before" Questionnaire

Copy the questions and your answers in your notebook, or download the Word document, and write your responses on the computer. *For your eyes only!*

Today's date ___________ Your current weight_______.

1. Family history of weight issues? Mother___________ Father___________ Siblings_____Other? ___________ Was weight a sore spot in the home? Do many of your close friends have weight issues?
2. How old were you when you first decided (or were told) you had a weight problem? _____
3. How much did you weigh at that time? _______ How did you feel about it?
4. List the diets, programs, and procedures you've tried in the past. What did you like/not like about each? What worked/didn't work about each? Do you recall why or what happened that led to your quitting each diet or program?
5. Did any of the things you've done make a lasting difference in your weight? In your self-image? What did, and in what way?
6. Did you ever think of yourself as being at your right weight? If so, when? If not, can you imagine yourself that way?
7. Do you think you are in touch with your body's hunger and fullness signals? Do you often eat when you aren't really hungry? Or eat to overfull? In what circumstances?

8. Do you mostly eat foods you love, or do you often feel you're sacrificing for your "regime?"
9. What are your current concerns besides losing weight? Circle those that apply: Health, alcohol, smoking, drugs, depression, loneliness, other. Elaborate on any that seem relevant to your weight.
10. Rate how you feel you're doing right now on a scale of 1 to 10 (sucky to great) in these areas of your life. Add comments if you wish.

    __ eating mostly nutritious foods

    __ getting regular exercise

    __ managing stress

    __ close relationships

    __ sufficient sleep

    __ energy level

    __ sex life

    __ mood

    __ productivity

    __ job satisfaction

    __ ability to speak up for yourself

    __ creative efforts

    __ recreation and fun

    __ self-esteem

    __ other

11. You have no doubt dealt successfully with many challenges and learning opportunities in your life (in business, sport, family life, hobbies, breaking bad habits or starting positive ones, etc.). What resources and skills can you bring forward from these experiences to serve as models for succeeding at this weight project? List them here.

    What kept you going when the going got tough?

12. What is the cost of doing nothing? If you made no changes in the way you have been eating (or dieting) and thinking about food, your weight and your

body, what would Future You be like? In a year? Ten years? How would you feel about yourself?

13. What are your goals for your weight mastery project (include attitude and behaviors as well as pounds)?

Chapter 5

Hunger Levels at Several Points During the Day

B% = Hunger Level ***Before*** eating **A%** = Hunger Level ***After*** eating

Time	B%	Situation	Sensations/Emotions?	A%	Notes

Observations at the end of the day:

Graphing Daily Hunger Levels

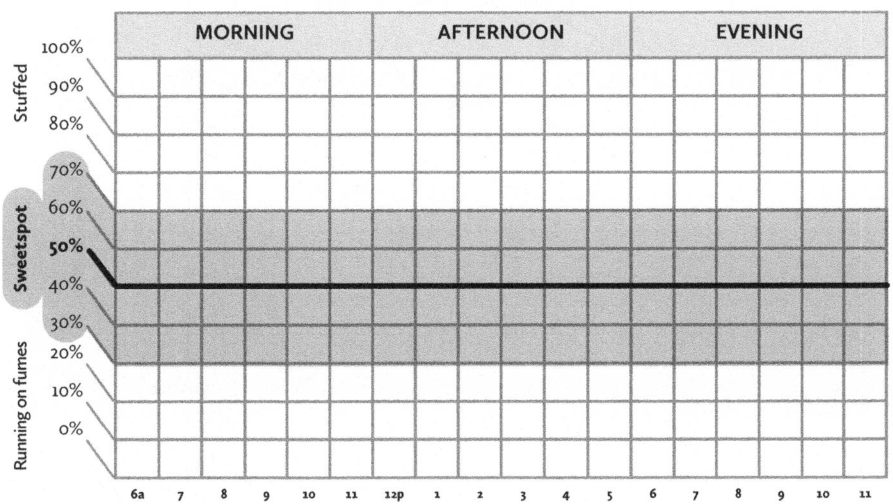

Observations at the end of the day:

Chapter 10

My Truthful Food Diary, Day, Date ____________

B% = Hunger Level ***Before*** eating **A%** = Hunger Level ***After*** eating

Time	B%	Place	Food/Amount	A%

Observations at the end of the day:

My Truthful Food Diary, with Reasons Day, Date ____________

B% = Hunger Level ***Before*** eating **A%** = Hunger Level ***After*** eating

Time	B%	Food/Amount	A%	Why I ate this

Observations at the end of the day:

Chapter 11: The Winning Formula and Daily Checklist

Make copies of the Winning Formula and post wherever you need to be reminded of them—especially on the door of the refrigerator or snack cabinet.

SuperTool #3: The Winning Formula

1. WAIT until you're hungry to eat—internal fuel gauge at 30% or below.
2. Take three deep breaths to center yourself before you eat. If you cannot relax enough to be present to your food and body, WAIT.
3. Sit down at a place set up for eating—not in your car, at your desk or on the couch.
4. Reduce distractions. No TV, radio, reading, or cell phone while you eat.
5. Slow down, so you can stay in communication with your internal fuel gauge.
6. Become aware of the sensory experience of eating the food.
7. If a food doesn't appeal to you, *don't eat it*.
8. STOP eating *before* you're full. Filling up to 70% on your inner fuel gauge is plenty.

An abridged "physical" version of the Winning Formula:

The Five-Point Checklist

Where to check (touch places in order):

GUT	Am I actually hungry? (Less than 30%)
PLACE	Am I sitting at a table in a calm environment?
HEAD	Am I centered and able to focus on eating?
MOUTH	Do I taste this food? Do I like it?
GUT	Have I had *just enough*? (No more than 70% full)

The Winning Formula Daily Checklist

Make check mark every time you follow that key.
Each box can have several checks since you eat several times a day.
At the end of the week look over the chart to see if you notice any patterns and record your observations.

The Winning Formula	Sun	Mon	Tues	Wed	Thurs	Fri	Sat
1 Wait till you're hungry to eat (fuel gauge at 30% or less)							
2 Take three breaths to center yourself							
3 Sit at a place set up for eating							
4 Reduce distractions (no TV, radio, cell phone, reading)							
5 Slow down and pay attention to your fuel gauge							
6 Be aware of all five senses as you eat							
7 If a food doesn't appeal to you, don't eat it							
8 Stop eating before you're full (fuel gauge at 70%)							

Observations at the end of the week:

Chapter 17: "Rate Your Food" Chart

Rate Your Food Chart

Rate from 1-10, 1=yuck, 5=passable, 10=fantastic

Name of food	Expectation	First bite	Last bite

Rate Your Food Chart

Rate from 1-10, 1=yuck, 5=passable, 10=fantastic

Name of food	Expectation	First bite	Last bite

Chapter 32: Snack Chart

My Moods and My Snacks

State of Mind	Example of Situation	My Go-To Snack	What I Could Do Instead
Overwhelmed			
Bored			
Tired			
Anxious, Worried			
Angry			
Procrastinating			
Indecision			
Lonely, Sad, Depressed			
Watching TV/Movies			
At Work			
Driving			
Happy, Content			
?			
?			

Observations:

Chapter 42 : "After" Questionnaire

The questions below are almost the same as on your "Before" form. Answer them after you've worked through the exercises in the book, but without referring back to your original answers.

Today's date_______

Best guess at your weight______ (because you tossed your scales)

1. Do you ever think of yourself as someone at their right size? If so, when? If not, can you imagine yourself as one?
2. Do you think you are in touch with your body's hunger and fullness signals? Do you often eat when you aren't really hungry? Or eat to overfull? In what circumstances?
3. Do you mostly eat foods you love or do you often feel you are sacrificing for your "regime?"
4. What are your current concerns besides losing weight? Circle those that apply: Health, alcohol, smoking, drugs, depression, loneliness, other. Elaborate on any that seem relevant to your weight.
5. Rate how you feel you are doing right now on a scale of 1 to 10 (sucky to great) in these areas of your life (feel free to add comments):

    __ eating mostly nutritious foods

    __ getting regular exercise

    __ managing stress

    __ close relationships

    __ sufficient sleep

    __ energy level

    __ sex life

    __ mood

    __ productivity

    __ job satisfaction

    __ ability to speak up for yourself

__ creative efforts

__ recreation and fun

__ self-esteem

__ other

Now refer back to your "Before" answers to compare. Then ask yourself:

- Have you been a Participant or a Spectator?
- Where do you see progress on your stated goal(s)?
- Where would you like to make some adjustments or improvements?
- What are the three most important behavior changes you've made since you started?
- What are the three most important attitude changes you've made?
- Have you acknowledged yourself for this progress?
- What is your plan of action going forward?
- Remember your *why*. You're completing this project so that you can ____________________.

APPENDIX B:
Guided Meditation Transcripts

All meditations can be found on a private page for readers
on my website: joyoverstreet.com/pie.
Please listen before reading.
Listening, rather than reading, bypasses your thinking mind.
It allows memories and images to pop up before you can judge them
or squash them as irrelevant. In order to make new discoveries,
your imagination needs the freedom to roam.

Chapter 4: Discovering Your Internal Fuel Gauge

Getting in touch with these sensations before, during, and after you eat is an essential awareness skill you're cultivating. Take your time between questions.

> Sit comfortably upright in a chair and, as you close your eyes, take three deep breaths… As you do, see if you can let go of the 10,000 things that are running around in your mind. You can pick them up later.…
>
> Now you're going to look through your body for any places you associate with hunger and fullness… In each location you're going to ask yourself the same question: are there any sensations there that you'd call hunger, time to eat, comfortable, full?
>
> Start with your mouth, teeth, and throat. Are there any sensations there that you'd call hunger, time to eat, comfortable, full?…
>
> When you think about or see food, do you experience any sensations in your hands that send you the message they want to grab something to eat?…

Move your attention to the stomach area, just below your rib cage. Are there any sensations there that you'd call hunger, time to eat, comfortable, full? How would you describe these sensations? Pinching, tightness, cramping, gassy, distended?...

Then focus on your abdomen. Are there any sensations there that you'd call hunger, time to eat, comfortable, full? How would you describe these sensations? Pinching, tightness, cramping, gassy, distended?...

After noting any sensations you associate with hunger or fullness, take your hands and feel the area of your abdomen and stomach. How do your clothes fit? (tight? loose? comfortable?)

Now imagine you've been blessed with an internal fuel gauge for your stomach that goes from 0 (running on fumes) to 100% (totally topped off)—with 50% being neither hungry nor full. At what hunger level (percentage from 0 to 100%) do you find yourself at this particular moment?

Repeat this fuel level check frequently until it becomes second nature.

Chapter 8: Me, Eating

Settle yourself into a comfortable seated position and uncross your arms and legs. As you allow your eyes to close, just let go of the countless things you had on your mind. You can pick them back up when we're done. Take your time between questions to let memories spring forth.

Take a deep breath… hold it… let it go with a big sigh. Again… One more time…

Now, get the idea that you are at the movies… You walk into a darkened theater and take a seat in your favorite section… feel the anticipation. The curtains roll back and you see the opening credits… and there's your name on the big screen! YOU are the star of this movie—in technicolor and surround sound.

The opening scene unfolds. And there you are, at your most recent meal. So now roll the clock back to the last time you ate. It could be last night's supper, today's lunch at your desk, a bagel at Starbucks…

*Where are you? And what are you eating?

What is going on in the environment around you?

Are you seated at a table set up specifically for eating?

Are you concentrating on your food or are you busy talking, checking email, or thinking about something else?

Were you hungry when you ate this food?

Now observe yourself eating this food: notice your method of eating, if it's fast or slow.

Do you ever have an empty mouth or put down your fork?

Do you taste the food?. .. Do you like what you're eating? Is it what you really want?

Now notice your emotional state. .. are you swallowing some unexpressed emotions along with the food?

When you're done with eating, how full are you? Are you feeling satisfied?

In sum, was this eating experience a pleasant or unpleasant one for you, and what made it that way?

Good job! Let that meal and its lessons fade from the screen. But don't get up yet. You've got one more scene to watch, because this is a double feature!

So now ***roll the clock back to the meal you had before the meal you just watched.*** If the memory that pops up is a different meal than the next to last one, go with that one. It's all good.

*Where are you? And what are you eating? (Repeat the questions from above.)

Well done! Let go of that meal and let the curtains close on the screen. Take a moment to feel your butt in the chair and your feet on the floor. Recall the room you're presently sitting in… and when you have a sense of being back in the present moment, you can open your eyes.

Take out your notebook and jot down your observations as in the prompt.

Chapter 9: You Have a Body

Standing Body Meditation

Remove your shoes and put down anything you might have in your hands. Find a place in the room where you can stand without being concerned about bumping into something when your eyes are shut. (If standing is a problem, you can also do this in a straight-back chair.) Give yourself time between questions to get the full experience.

Stand with your feet slightly apart, and rock back and forth until you feel well-grounded. Now close your eyes and do a quick head-to-toe scan.

Do any areas of your body feel uncomfortable or tense? If so, see if you can wiggle them a bit looser.

Now pay attention to your breathing. Take three slow breaths as follows:

Breathing in, I calm my body. Breathing out, let go of fear.

Breathing in, deep relaxation. Breathing out, my mind is clear.

Breathing in, this perfect moment. Breathing out, I'm present, here.

With your eyes closed, become aware of your feet. Are you gripping with your toes? Notice where your weight is balanced by shifting a little to the right, to the left, toward your toes, toward your heels. Where is your normal balance point?

As you pay attention to your feet, is there any discomfort? Do you have any attitudes or judgments about your feet? What about your ankles?

Now, become aware of your calves. What sensations do you feel in your calves? Do you notice how they help keep your balance? What attitudes and evaluations do you have about your calves? Reach down and feel your ankles and calves. Give them a kindly pat.

Notice your knees. Are they locked? Do you feel any sensations in your knees? What attitudes and evaluations do you have about your knees? Reach down and give your knees a little massage.

Move your attention to your upper legs and thighs. Do you notice any tensions there? What attitudes and evaluations do you have about your upper legs and thighs? Good. Use your hands to feel your upper legs and thighs. All the way around. Notice if they feel the same as, better, or worse than you thought they did.

Now focus on the area of your hips and buttocks. What sensations do you notice in your hips and buttocks? Are you gripping with your butt? What attitudes, emotions, and evaluations do you have about your hips and buttocks? Fine. Use your hands to feel your hips and buttocks. Notice if they feel the same as, better, or worse than you thought they did.

Move your attention now to the area of your stomach, abdomen, and waist. Do you feel any sensations there? Are your abdominal muscles pulled in tight, or are you letting it all hang out? Is that your normal state? Notice if you're feeling hungry, or just right, or full. What attitudes, emotions, and evaluations do you have about your stomach, abdomen, and waist? Take your time here. Use your hands to feel your stomach, your abdomen, your waist. Do these parts feel like you thought they would? Better? Worse?

Now focus your attention on the area of your chest, breasts, and rib cage, feeling the rise and fall of your chest as you breathe. Is your breathing shallow? Deep? Do you feel your rib cage expand? What attitudes, emotions, and evaluations do you have about your chest, breasts, and rib cage? Use your hands to feel your chest, your breasts, and your rib cage. What do you notice now?

Release your arms to hang at your sides. How do they feel? Are they comfortable? Are your hands loosely open? What attitudes and evaluations do you have about your arms and hands? Using the opposite hand, feel each arm and hand.

Now become aware of your shoulders and the area at the back of your neck. Can you let your shoulders fall a little lower? Is there tension between your shoulder blades or in your neck? Roll your shoulders back and forth, up and down. Turn your head from side to side, then up and down, to loosen your neck.

Now focus your awareness on your face. What sensations do you have in your face? Are you frowning? Clamping your jaw? See if you can let your jaw drop. Use your hands to feel your face as if you've never felt it before. Feel the area under your chin. What attitudes and evaluations do you have about your face, your neck, your chin? Now reach up to the top of your head and give your hair a gentle fluffing as you massage your scalp.

OK. Observing your body as a whole, at this moment, what part of your body do you like the most? OK. At this moment, what part do you like the least? Was it hard to touch that part? Can you allow yourself to accept that part as it is, just for now?

Can you bring yourself to give yourself a hug? This is the perfect moment to do that.

Before you open your eyes, recall the room you're standing in and the furniture that's around you. Take a couple of deep breaths, and once again feel your feet on the floor. When your mind is back in the room, open your eyes. Nicely done!

Take out your notebook and write down what you noticed, per the prompt.

Chapter 14: "I Did it Myself!"

Seat yourself in a comfortable chair, uncross your arms and legs and close your eyes.

Gently nod your head yes, and shake your head no. Let your jaw unclench and that space between your eyebrows loosen. Good.

Now take three centering breaths with me:

> *Breathing in I calm my body; breathing out doubt and fear*
>
> *Breathing in deep relaxation; breathing out, my mind is clear*
>
> *Breathing in this perfect moment; being fully present here.*

Go back in your memory and see if you can pinpoint the time you began to get fat, or first believed you had a weight problem.

> *When was this? How old were you? What happened?*
>
> *If you're drawing a blank, just recall the most recent time you gained a bunch of weight.*

Now let's pretend, that right from the get-go, you planned it all out. As preposterous as this sounds, pretend you made a decision to gain weight. You figured it out and methodically carried out the plan…

> *What are you doing? What's your process and how is it working out? What else did you do?*

Now get the idea that this fat or this weight problem has been useful to you in some way.

> *How has it been useful?*
>
> *What has it protected you from?*
>
> *If this feels too close to the bone, imagine what someone else would do to get fat—why would they do that?*

Let go of these images and gradually bring your attention back to your body in the chair. Take a few deep breaths and open your eyes. Nicely done!

Grab your notebook and jot down your observations, per the prompt.

Chapter 20: Your "True Thin" Friends

Set aside at least fifteen minutes to do this meditation and write up your observations. As you bring these people to mind, you may wonder if the person is really a true thin, or just putting on a good show. It doesn't matter. Just take the images you get.

Get yourself into a comfortable position seated in a chair. Uncross your arms and legs and close your eyes. Take a deep breath... hold it... let it go with a big sigh. Again...

> *Now, bring to mind a slim friend or acquaintance—not a fat person hiding in a thin body, but someone you believe to be a true thin from the inside... Understand that people without weight worries come in many guises and sizes; just take whoever pops into your mind.
>
> Bring to mind an incident in which the friend was with some food...
>
> > *What are they eating (or not eating)?*
> >
> > *How are they eating—fast, slow, with interest or disinterest?*
> >
> > *What do they eat first? Last?*
> >
> > *Do they toy with their food or rearrange it on the plate? Do they leave any behind?*
> >
> > *How do they seem to relate to the food? Any attitudes you notice?*
> >
> > *What kind of person is this friend? Do you have certain judgments about him or her? Do you like this person?*
>
> Let that friend go and open your eyes.

In your notebook, jot down your observations. Repeat the meditation from *above with a different friend (as many times as you find helpful).

Chapter 21: The Wall Comes Down

Settle yourself into a comfortable seated position, arms uncrossed, feet flat on the floor. Keep your notebook nearby, but don't have anything on your lap. As you let your eyes gently close, allow yourself to drop the countless things swirling in your mind. Give yourself plenty of time between suggestions to let the images emerge. Whatever you get is perfect.

> Take a minute now to go through your body and notice any tensions you may be feeling. Are you frowning? Clenching your jaw? Rotate your head from side to side, then up and down to loosen your neck...
>
> We'll take three deep breaths together now:
>
> > *Breathing in, I calm my body. Breathing out, let go of fear.*
> >
> > *Breathing in, deep relaxation. Breathing out, my mind is clear.*
> >
> > *Breathing in, this perfect moment. Breathing out, I'm present, here...*
>
> Now imagine yourself out in a beautiful open space. It could be at the beach, or in a meadow, in a soaring cathedral, on a mountaintop. Whatever image comes is fine. Take time to see this beautiful space... to feel the sun on your back, to hear a gentle wind blowing... maybe birdsong, music, waves. To smell the pine needles or salt air or flowers... Just enjoy BEing in this space. Peaceful and content...
>
> Now get the idea that you are a just-right-sized person, your most perfect self (however you envision that person to be), looking exactly the way you want to look, feeling exactly the way you want to feel... standing, sitting, or lying in this beautiful open space.
>
> To make this self really real to you, without opening your eyes, bring your hands into the air in front of you and begin creating your perfect body as a sculptor might. Nobody's watching, so make these gestures large and expressive.

Start at the head… don't forget your nose, your ears, your hair.

Your shoulders… your upper torso… your arms… your hands.

Now your waist and hips. Don't forget your back side!

Your legs… your feet. What shoes are you wearing? Or are you barefoot?

Now stand back and make sure you are exactly the way you want to be… Are there any finishing touches you want to add?

Now see yourself as this perfect just-right-sized person moving… doing things… walking proudly down the street… maybe dancing… making love… happy, free… feeling really good about your body… appreciating how it supports your purpose.

…

Now imagine that you've created a wall that surrounds this perfect vision of yourself… But this is no ordinary wall—it's made of everything you associate with your weight problem—foods, for sure, but so much more.

Without opening your eyes, use your hands out in front of you to build this wall. Stack it with every sort of food you want to pile on: heaps and blobs of French fries, cottage cheese, donuts, chips 'n' dip, sugar-free cookies, celery sticks, Snickers bars, fat-free ice cream, hot fudge sundaes… You might want to extend the wall to your right and left as well. Pack it and stack it!

What else? anything else?… Very nice!

But wait! We're not done. This is a very special wall, made up of a lot more than food.

Bring to mind some people you'd like to shove into the wall, head or feet first…, your ex-partner, your mean third grade teacher, your mom, a co-worker, the boss who harassed you, your stepfather, a playground bully, a sibling… All the people who have hurt you get stuck into this wall… Those awful things they said or did to you… stick those memories in the wall too.

This special wall even includes thoughts and emotions… As feelings are coming up for you, pluck them out of your head and slap them on the wall. Pull those arrows from your heart and shove them into the wall too…

How about some tired old beliefs and excuses? Poke those into any chinks you see...

Wow! Great job! Now stand back and take a good look at this wall you've created. How big is it? How solid? Does it have a texture? A smell?

…

Now get the idea the wall can communicate with your perfect self… what would it want to tell you?

What else does it want to say to you? Anything else? Notice your emotions as you listen to it…

Now get the idea you can talk to the wall so it really gets what you're saying… what would you tell the wall? It's OK to yell. It's OK to cry.

What else do you want to tell it? Anything else?

Notice how you feel as you express yourself fully. Well done...

Now, thank your wall for all it's done for you over these many years… how it's been a protector, a friend, a buffer.

You have one more question for your wall. Ask it: What's on the other side?… and let it answer…

Then ask yourself this important question: What have I walled out?… and *who* have I walled out?

…

You are so ready to be DONE with this wall! But keep your eyes shut.

Tell the wall you're going to destroy it, and notice the emotions and sensations that arise…

Now, using any means that come to mind, destroy the wall. Use dynamite, fire or fire hoses, roto-rooters, backhoes, hungry lions, shovels and pitchforks—have at it!

As the wall comes down, again notice your emotions and sensations…

And there you are! Your healthy right-sized self, revealed. You're free, once again out in that beautiful open space. Allow yourself to run, dance, hop or just sit there and breathe…

Get the idea that you can bring your perfect self back to the room with you… take your time.

Take a few deep breaths… feel your feet on the floor… your butt in the chair… and open your eyes.

When you're back in the room, before you do anything else, get out your notebook and write what you noticed in the meditation, as well as whatever else comes up for you—connections, other memories.

Chapter 25: Affirming Your Ideal Self

Set aside several minutes where you won't be disturbed, and have your notebook nearby so you can take notes when we're done. Your job is to let the images and words wash over you. Don't worry if you find yourself arguing with every phrase. That's your resistance talking. We will deal with that in the next part of the book. Later you can write your own affirmations and record them on the voice memo app on your smart phone.

Seat yourself in a comfortable chair and close your eyes.

Let's take three deep breaths together and as you do, let go of the 10,000 things running around in your mind:

Breathing in, I calm my body. Breathing out, let go of fear.

Breathing in, deep relaxation. Breathing out, my mind is clear.

Breathing in, this perfect moment. Breathing out, I'm present, here.

Take yourself back to the image you created of your perfect self as you stepped outside that wall you built and destroyed. There you are in that beautiful open space, feeling light and free. Watch yourself sway, move, dance…

As I say each positive statement, I'll pause for a moment to let you repeat the line to yourself and see how it feels. There's no right or wrong way to do this. If resistance comes up, just notice it and continue. No big deal.

I am the master of my eating.

I'm at peace with food and free of its spell.

I slowly savor my food, grateful for the pleasure it brings.

I am attracted to foods that improve my health.

I eat when I'm sitting down in a calm environment.

I eat only when I'm physically hungry.

I recognize when I've eaten just enough and simply stop eating.

I feel good about stopping before I'm full.

I eat selectively, only those foods that appeal to me.

I love to awaken my palate with new foods and new cuisines.

I enjoy the power of leaving food on my plate.

I am stronger than a bag of potato chips, more powerful than fudge.

At parties I focus on getting to know other people, not the buffet.

I can say "No, thank you," without feeling the least bit guilty.

I can throw food away without pangs of attachment.

I can leave my tired excuses behind.

I appreciate this miraculous body I've been given.

I treat my body with love and compassion.

I'm the only me in the whole world, so I carry myself with pride.

I have many skillful ways to deal with my feelings besides eating.

I am the master of my eating.

I'm at peace with food and my body.

Feel your feet on the floor, and your butt in the chair, and slowly come back to the room…

Make some notes on what you observed and discovered.

Chapter 36: The Apologies and Appreciation Tour

Give yourself time between each suggestion. Take off your shoes so you can ground yourself through your feet. Stand or seat yourself in a comfortable chair, then close your eyes.

Let's take three deep breaths together, to help you let go of all the thoughts running around in your mind:

Breathing in, I calm my body. Breathing out, let go of fear.

Breathing in, deep relaxation. Breathing out, my mind is clear.

Breathing in, this grateful moment. Breathing out, I'm present, here.

As you center yourself, take yourself back to that vision of yourself in the beautiful open space you created after you destroyed your custom-built wall. See yourself—happy, free, dancing, loving and loved…

With that loving state of mind, become aware of your feet. Wiggle them, flex them. Think about what they do for you every day, ever since you were a toddler, carrying you from here to there, especially those times when you've crammed them into painful shoes… or burdened them with too many pounds. Feel your feet with your hands. Apologize for your unkind thoughts and actions. Experience a wave of gratitude for them…

With a loving state of mind, become aware of your ankles, lower legs, and knees. Wiggle them, flex them. Think about what they do for you every day, carrying you from here to there, especially those times when you've burdened them with too many pounds. Feel your lower legs and knees with your hands. Apologize for your unkind thoughts and actions. Experience a wave of gratitude for them…

With a loving state of mind, become aware of your thighs and hips. Wiggle them, shake them. Think about what they do for you every day, carrying you from here to there, especially those times when you've insulted them, squeezed them into too-tight garments, wishing they would disappear. Feel your thighs and hips with your hands. Apologize for your unkind thoughts and actions. Experience a wave of gratitude…

With a loving state of mind, become aware of your butt. Wiggle it, shake it. Think about what it does for you every day, cushioning you from the pain of hard seats, perhaps attracting potential sexual partners, helping you pull off dance moves. Have you wished your butt would disappear? Feel your butt with your hands. Apologize for your unkind thoughts and actions. Send it grateful thoughts…

With a loving state of mind, become aware of your back. Arch it like a cow, curve it like a cat. Stretch it from side to side. Gently twist to the right and then to the left. Think about what your back does for you every day, holding you upright, keeping you from being a spineless blob. Have you ignored your back (except when it hurts)? Feel your back with your hands. Apologize for your unkind thoughts and actions. Send it grateful thoughts…

With a loving state of mind, become aware of your stomach and abdominal area. Repeat the arching, curving, stretching, twisting motions you did for your back. You can't move one without the other. Think about what goes on inside your stomach and abdomen every day! All those organs in there that transform what you eat into fuel to keep you going! Feel your stomach and abdominal area with your hands. Apologize for your many unkind thoughts and actions. Experience a wave of gratitude for them…

While you're appreciating what's inside your trunk, become aware of all the reproductive organs that keep the human species going. The miracle of sex—and if you are female— pregnancy, birth, and lactation. Experience a wave of gratitude for them…

With a loving state of mind, become aware of your lungs. Take three more slow deep breaths and let your chest rise and fall. Do you remember to breathe often enough? Do you take your lungs outside so they can breathe the fresh air? The breath is life—the life force. Without oxygen we die. The word inspiration means breath. Apologize for ignoring your lungs and the gift of your breath. Breathe in your gratitude for your lungs.

With a loving state of mind, become aware of your shoulders, arms and hands. Shrug your shoulders—up, up, up, then let them drop. Do it again. Now give your arms and hands a shake. Rotate your wrists and flex them forward and back. Nice. Think about what they do for you every day, lifting, carrying heavy loads, using all manner of tools to improve your life, including the fork with which you feed yourself, the computer and pen you use to write. They do the finest of manipulations. With each hand, feel the opposite shoulder, arm and hand. Apologize to them for any unkind thoughts and actions. Let yourself experience a wave of gratitude for them.

With a loving state of mind, become aware of your head and neck. Turn your head slowly from side to side. Rotate your head down, to the right, to the back, to the left and back to center. Repeat in the other direction. Open your mouth wide, stick out your tongue, and hiss like an angry cat. Feel your face... your skin, your eyes, your nose, your mouth, your chin. Scritch your scalp as if you were washing your hair. Think about all that your head is doing for you—your brain is stuffed with ideas, stories, memories, dreams, practical know-how. And your neck has to hold all of it up! Apologize to your head and neck for your lack of appreciation and any insults you may have hurled at them. Let yourself experience a wave of gratitude for them.

This body of yours may not meet with your exacting standards—you are not Beyoncé, you are not elegant Amal Clooney, you are not Arnold Schwarzenegger, and you never will be. You have aches, pains, sags and bags. Nevertheless, at this very moment realize that *you are a miracle*!

How can you not be devoted to the loving care of this body of yours? It's time to stop treating your body like it was a rental car.

We will close with some affirmations

My body is my friend and constant companion.

I treat my body with the respect it deserves.

I appreciate the feet and legs that take me where I want to go.

I appreciate my soft butt that cushions me when I sit.

I marvel at all the organs in my trunk that keep me nourished.

I marvel at my lungs that fill me with the breath of life.

I appreciate my arms and hands for their constant efforts to do my bidding.

I am filled with wonder that I can see, taste, smell, feel, think, and love.

I care for my body as if it were my most precious possession.

I honor my body by feeding it the quality food it deserves.

I am attracted to foods that improve my health.

I honor my body by eating just enough and never too much.,

I honor my body by exercising it in some way every day.

I appreciate this miraculous body I've been given.

I'm the only me in the world, so I carry myself with pride.

Now, thank your body from the bottom of your heart, and give yourself a big bear hug. Gradually bring your attention back to the room. Feel your feet on the floor and open your eyes. Repeat any time you feel out of sorts with your body.

Chapter 42: My Healthy Beloved Body

In our final meditation, we'll connect you again with your precious body, and we'll conclude with affirmations. Seat yourself in a comfortable chair, uncross your arms and legs and close your eyes. Pause between instructions to give your mind time to come up with the images.

> Let's take three deep breaths together and as you do, let go of the 10,000 things running around in your mind:
>
> *Breathing in, I calm my body. Breathing out, let go of fear.*
>
> *Breathing in, deep relaxation. Breathing out, my mind is clear.*
>
> *Breathing in, this perfect moment. Breathing out, I'm present, here.*
>
> Visualize yourself as you are right now, and breathe deeply into your center—that area just below your naval… Create a feeling of warmth and strength in that center…
>
> Allow that feeling of warmth and strength to radiate outwards, then upward through your rib cage, up your spine to your shoulders.
>
> Feel the warmth and strength running out your arms to your hands… and up your neck to the top of your head. And now down your legs all the way to your feet.
>
> Now get the idea that this warmth and strength has the power to melt away all your negative self-images… Visualize those hurtful thoughts getting mushy and so soft they melt into a clear orange liquid...
>
> Now imagine you have a drain plug at the end of your left big toe. You open the spigot and the orange liquid flows out and into a drain in the floor. You are doing this with your own warmth and strength.
>
> As the melted negativity flows out, you begin to sense your body with increasing clarity and appreciation. So stand back and look

yourself over, top to toe, front to back. Admire your body's sturdy persistence and its skill at keeping you alive.

Now imagine you can have a conversation with your body... Ask your body what it wants to tell you… and listen.

What else does it want to say to you?

Your turn: what would you like to tell your body? Speak it.

Remind your body that you are partners in this endeavor called life, and you are devoted to its well-being.

Give it a big bear hug.

Keep your eyes closed and repeat after me these affirmations to yourself:

I am the master of my eating.

I'm at peace with food and free of its spell.

I slowly savor my food, grateful for the pleasure it brings.

I am attracted to foods that improve my health.

I eat when I'm sitting down in a calm environment.

I eat only when I'm physically hungry.

I recognize when I've eaten just enough and simply stop eating.

I feel good about stopping before I'm full.

I eat selectively, only those foods that appeal to me.

I love to awaken my palate with new foods and new cuisines.

I enjoy the power of leaving food on my plate.

I am stronger than a bag of potato chips, more powerful than fudge.

At parties I focus on getting to know other people, not the buffet.

I can say "No, thank you," without feeling the least bit guilty.

I can throw food away without pangs of attachment.

I can leave my tired excuses behind.

I appreciate this miraculous body I've been given.

I treat my body with love and compassion.

I'm the only me in the whole world, so I carry myself with pride.

I have many skillful ways to deal with my feelings besides eating.

I am the master of my eating.

I'm at peace with food and my body.

Gradually get a sense of your butt in the chair, your feet on the floor, and the room you are in. And when you're back here, you can open your eyes.

APPENDIX C:
Resources
[books, articles, credits, websites]

Here you'll find sources for quotes and the books I've used for background material, organized by chapter. I've commented on ones I think are worth seeking out for yourself.

Opening quote by Shōma Morita, M.D. Morita was a well-known Japanese psychiatrist and contemporary of Sigmund Freud. Not surprisingly, due to his Zen Buddhist background, Morita's healing methods focused on paying attention, accepting reality and one's feelings as is, and taking constructive action anyway. In the United States, Morita's teachings continue, thanks to Gregg Krech at the TōDō Institute (http://www.todoinstitute.com), David K. Reynolds of Constructive Living, and others.

Introduction

Back in 1975, Chérie Carter-Scott was sharpening her innovative vocational coaching techniques on me. She participated in one of my very first Thin Within workshop series, so you could say we were guinea pigs for each other. Today she is known as the "mother of life coaching." Her business, The MMS Institute, offers leadership and coach-training services around the world.

"True thins and fat thins": I finally tracked down the source of this brilliant concept to the same Dr. Theodore Isaac Rubin, whose harsh assessment of anyone carrying a few extra pounds as "sick" so pained me ("Fatness is a sickness" in chapter 1). In his book, *Forever Thin* (New York: Gramercy Publishing, 1970), he describes the differences between how an "obese" person relates to food versus how a "true thin" does, noting that even at "normal" weight, the obese person will always be in the grip of diet mentality. Where Rubin and I differ is that he believed that the obese mindset was incurable. I know from experience that the "true thin" mind-set, once uncovered, can be strengthened and with practice, become permanent.

The humanist psychologist Abraham Maslow rejected the psychiatric tradition of focusing on people's troubled pasts. Instead, he believed that people already possess the inner resources for growth and healing, so therapy should help them remove obstacles to experiencing their wholeness. https://en.wikipedia.org/wiki/Abraham_Maslow.

Journaling is a powerful tool for self-discovery. Although her famous book, *The Artist's Way*, is focused on unleashing your creativity, Julia Cameron's daily journaling process and ideas are a model for how to use a notebook to wake up your dormant selves. Julia Cameron, *The Artist's Way: A Spiritual Path to Higher Creativity* (New York: Tarcher/Putnam, 1992).

Chapter 1: Coming to Terms with the F-Word

"Fatness is a sickness": Theodore Isaac Rubin, M.D, *The Thin Book by a Formerly Fat Psychiatrist* (New York: Simon and Schuster, 1966). Not recommended

Chapter 3: Is Your Weight Your Fault?

"America's love affair with dieting": Fad diets and weight loss have a long history, going back to the mid-1800s. In the early 20th century, international food shortages around World War I led the U.S. government to promote eating less and being thin as patriotic. Those who were overweight were seen as somehow morally deficient. The books below are real eye-openers. Have we made progress? Not sure.

"Lay your double chin on the altar of liberty": Helen Zoe Veit, *Modern Food, Moral Food: Self Control, Science, and the Rise of Modern American Eating in the Early Twentieth Century* (Chapel Hill, University of North Carolina Press, 2013).

Susan Yager, *The Hundred Year Diet, America's Voracious Appetite for Losing Weight* (New York: Rodale, 2010).

"Since the birth of farming": Bee Wilson, *The Way We Eat Now: How the Food Revolution Has Transformed Our Lives, Our Bodies, and Our World* (New York: Basic Books, 2019).

"Food feels dangerous": Virginia Sole-Smith, *The Eating Instinct: Food Culture, Body Image, and Guilt in America* (New York: Henry Holt & Co., 2018) If you're raising kids this is a must read.

Eric Schlosser, *Fast Food Nation* (New York: Houghton Mifflin, 2001).

Chapter 4: What Is Your Responsibility?

Lindy West, *Shrill*. (New York: Hachette Books, 2016).

Chapter 5: Calibrating your Eyes

Brian Wansink, *Mindless Eating, Why We Eat More Than We Think We Do* (New York: Bantam Books, 2007).

Chapter 6: Calibrating Your Fuel Gauge

Evelyn Tribole and Elaine Resch, *Intuitive Eating: A Revolutionary Anti-Diet Approach*, 4th Edition (New York: St. Martin's Essentials, 2020). The authors' philosophy and practices align closely with my own. They cite current scientific studies that back up what we figured out experientially at Thin Within back in the 1970s. If you need continuing support on your anti-diet journey, check them out at www.intuitiveeating.org.

Annie Murphy Paul, *The Extended Mind: The Power of Thinking Outside the Brain*, (Boston: Houghton Mifflin Harcourt, 2021). Tuning up your interoceptive awareness has many surprising benefits, as do my other body awareness exercises. She explains why, and backs it up with scientific research.

Chapter 7: Square One

"Part of getting to know yourself": Lori Gottlieb, *Maybe You Should Talk to Someone* (New York: Houghton Mifflin Harcourt, 2019). An intriguing exploration by a therapist who is also in therapy herself. Her 2019 TEDTalk, "How Changing Your Story Can Change Your Life," brilliantly describes the power of our personal narratives.

Chapter 9: You Have a Body

"Rule 1. You will receive a body": Excerpted from *If Life Is a Game, These Are the Rules: Ten Rules For Being Human As Introduced In Chicken Soup For The Soul* by Chérie Carter-Scott, © 1998. Used by permission of Broadway Books, an imprint of Random House, a division of Penguin Random House LLC. All rights reserved.

Chapter 11: The Winning Formula

"Breathing in": Veronika Noize is the DIY Marketing Coach and leader of a thriving support community I've been part of since 2005. She can be found here: https://www.diymarketingcenter.com.

"Neuroscience tells us": David B. Eagleman, *Livewired: The Inside Story of the Ever-Changing Brain* (New York: Pantheon, 2020).

"Wait until you're hungry to eat": Alan Dolit, *Fat Liberation* (Millbrae: Celestial Arts, 1975). Dolit's obscure but groundbreaking book of eating awareness exercises may have been the first to use a checklist for eating more consciously.

Chapter 12: Negativity Bias

"Your brain is like velcro": Rick Hanson, Ph.D., *Buddha's Brain* (Oakland: New Harbinger Publications, 2009). Hanson has written extensively about the neuroplasticity of the brain and how it can be shaped through mindfulness, since your brain learns mainly from what you attend to. A useful perspective.

Chapter 13: Don't Call Me a Machine!

In 1970, Werner Erhard created the hugely popular and widely imitated human potential training program known as **est** (sometimes called Erhard Seminars Training) in San Francisco. Soon after my husband was diagnosed with cancer, he and I took the **est** training because we knew we needed better tools to navigate the uncertain times ahead.

est is actually Latin for ***it is*** because the goal of this very Zen program was to wake you up to the reality of the present moment—*it is what it is*. Recognizing that, we now have a choice of what to do with it. It's hard to describe the profound shift in perspective this realization unleashes.

It changed my life. In fact, the original Thin Within program reflected my interpretation of *est* as applied to weight "problems." I believe that if you *actually do the work* of this book, you too will experience a lasting shift—a transformation—in your relationship to food, your weight, and your body.

Currently a much kinder, gentler version of **est**, the *Landmark Forum*, still trains thousands of people a year around the world. I recommend it. https://www.landmarkworldwide.com.

Adelaide Bry, *est: 60 hours that transform your life* (New York: Avon Books, 1975). It's out of print but remains a fair representation of the program at the time I participated.

"Argue for your limitations": Richard Bach, *Jonathan Livingston Seagull* (New York: Scribner, 1970) This is a perennial bestselling fable about a seagull with aspirations.

Chapter 14: Standards—The Shoulds and the Shouldn'ts

"Shame contributes measurably": Lindy West, *Shrill.* (New York: Hachette Books, 2016).

"For some reason, we are truly convinced": Geneen Roth, *Women Food and God: An Unexpected Path to Almost Everything* (New York: Scribner, 2010). Geneen was one of my Thin Within students back in the late 1970s. She has gone on to spread the gospel of a mindful, compassionate, diet-free path to a healthier relationship with food and the body. Her retreats, online workshops, and her beautifully written books are an inspiration to many. Recommended. Find more at her website, www.geneenroth.com.

Chapter 17: Rate Your Food

"Fascinating new research in neuroscience": Lisa Feldman Barrett, *How Emotions are Made: The Secret Life of the Brain.* (Boston: Houghton Mifflin Harcourt, 2017). Barrett describes an eating experience she contrived for her daughter's birthday party, where she used the appearance of various foods to trick the partygoers' tastebuds. This book really made me think.

PART FOUR

Carol Dweck, *Mindset: The New Psychology of Success* (New York: Ballantine Books, 2007). Useful if you are interested in the research behind "growth mindset."

Chapter 19: The Cycle of Self-Fulfilling Prophecies

"Be-Do-Have": Werner Erhard, *the est training*, 1972

James Clear, in his mega-bestseller, *Atomic Habits* (New York: Avery Penguin Random House, 2018) describes how identity drives behavior and outcomes. His depiction of Be-Do-Have as three concentric circles is very helpful.

Chapter 20: What is Goal-Mindset?

"copy-and-paste": Katy Milkman, *How to Change: The Science of Getting from Where You Are to Where You Want to Be* (New York, Penguin/Portfolio, 2021). Buttress my book's tools with hers. Recommended.

Chapter 26: Positive Programming

"Affirmations were popularized by": Shakti Gawain, *Creative Visualization: Use the Power of Your Imagination to Create What You Want in Your Life* (Novato: New World Library, 2016). Although this book has been out since 1978, the message is still relevant; most books about the "law of attraction" are based on Gawain's work. She describes in detail how to create and use affirmations for all aspects of your life. She also connects them with the Be ➤ Do ➤ Have model I describe in Chapter 19.

Chapter 27: Teaser or Pleaser? SuperTool #5

"Teaser or Pleaser:" Leonard Pearson, MD, *The Psychologist's Eat-Anything Diet.* (New York, P.H. Wyden, 1973). Pearson was way ahead of his time. His words for "teasers and pleasers" were "beckoners and hummers." Same idea.

"sparks joy": Marie Kondo, *The Life-Changing Magic of Tidying Up* and *Spark Joy* (Berkeley: Ten Speed Press, 2016). Kondo is definitely worth a read if you also suffer from clutter problems. Extra pounds and extra stuff often go hand in hand. Attachment to our stuff is not that different from attachment to our food.

Chapter 28: Speaking of Cottage Cheese

Alan Lakein, *How to Get Control of Your Time and Your Life.* (New York, Signet, 1973). Lakein was the original time management guru. His famous question: "What is the best use of my time right now?" is no less relevant today than it was decades ago. Still an excellent book.

Chapter 29: Your Kitchen—Friend or Foe

"You don't have to be the victim": James Clear, *Atomic Habits* p. 30.

Since you're reading my book because your eating and/or thinking habits have been leading you astray, consider two other great books on habit change:

Gretchen Rubin, *Better Than Before* (New York: Broadway Books, 2015). I particularly love how she categorizes the different strategies you might need to use for specific problems. Her concept of loopholes is quite similar to the Pirates I describe in chapter 31: "Mutiny on the Bounty." My only disagreement with her is her devotion to a keto diet. It works for her all-in "upholder" personality. Otherwise her book is terrific.

Charles Duhigg, *The Power of Habit: Why We Do What We Do in Life and Business* (New York: Random House, 2014).

Chapter 30: Cue the Negative Pushback

"what Byron Katie calls The Work": Byron Katie, *Loving What Is: Four Questions that Can Change Your Life* (New York: Three Rivers Press, 2002), 19. *Loving What Is* describes her powerful process in detail with lots of examples of how she uses it with real people with real problems. If you're feeling stuck, especially in relationships, I suggest you watch some of her many free YouTube videos (https://www.youtube.com/user/TheWorkofBK). Her website, https://thework.com, offers free downloads of her worksheets and instructions.

Chapter 32: Snack Attack!

"the proliferation of snack foods": Michael Moss, *Salt Sugar Fat: How the Food Giants Hooked Us* (New York: Random House, 2014). Also *Hooked*, (New York: Random House, 2021). Our addiction to these ingredients is no accident. His award-winning books may make you angry enough you swear off snacks for good.

"the discomfort that precedes a snack attack": Nir Eyal, *Indistractable: How to Control Your Attention and Choose Your Life* (Dallas: BenBellaBooks, 2019)

"As you find yourself reaching for a snack": Judson Brewer, a psychiatrist and neuroscientist, has written two excellent books on changing mental habits, like snacking and anxiety: *The Craving Mind: From Cigarettes to Smartphones to Love—Why We Get Hooked and How we Can Break Bad Habits* (New Haven: Yale University Press, 2017) and *Unwinding Anxiety: New Science Shows How to Break the Cycles of Worry and Fear to Heal Your Mind* (New York: Avery, 2021). Highly recommended. His smart phone apps, *Eat Right Now* and *Unwinding Anxiety* are worth exploring.

Chapter 33: Be Like a Rocket

"Your outcomes are a lagging measure": James Clear, *Atomic Habits*, p. 18

Chapter 34: The Pigout Party

"disenchantment has set in": Judson Brewer's ideas about being "enchanted by" the addictive substance, and his process of experiencing it fully are very similar to mine. Back in the 1970s I had no scientific studies to prove the efficacy of taste-testing and rating the food—I just knew it worked. He's done the research and discusses it in his books, above.

Chapter 36: Other People

If you're a parent with young children, read these two books!

Bee Wilson, *First Bite, How We Learn to Eat* (New York: Basic Books, 2016).

Virginia Sole-Smith, *The Eating Instinct: Food Culture, Body Image, and Guilt in America.*

Chapter 38: Nutrition and Exercise Do Matter

"Eat food. Not too much. Mostly plants.": Michael Pollan, *In Defense of Food: An Eater's Manifesto* (New York: Penguin Books, 2009).

"Don't eat anything your grandmother wouldn't recognize as food.": Michael Pollan, *Food Rules, An Eater's Manual* (New York: Penguin Books, 2009).

"5-4-3-2-1 Go!": Mel Robbins, *The 5-Second Rule: Transform Your Life, Work and Confidence with Everyday Courage* (Savio Republic, 2017).

Chapter 39: Plateaus and the Plague of Perfectionism

"As beautifully as Yo-Yo Ma plays": Martin Steinberg, "Yo-Yo Ma on Intonation, Practice, and the Role of Music in Our Lives," *Strings*, September 17, 2015, https://stringsmagazine.com/yo-yo-ma-on-intonation-practice-and-the-role-of-music-in-our-lives.

Dan Harris' popular weekly podcast, *Ten Percent Happier*, is really terrific. He is an engaging host and his guests are always topnotch. He also has a meditation app by the same name. Start with his book, *10% Happier Revised Edition: How I Tamed the Voice in My Head, Reduced Stress Without Losing My Edge, and Found Self-Help That Actually Works—A True Story.* (Dey Street Book, 2019)

Chapter 42: Life Is a Game

"Life is a game.": Werner Erhard, *Up to Your Ass in Aphorisms.* (San Francisco: **est**, 1973.)

William Bridges, *Transitions: Making Sense of Life's Changes*, 2nd edition (DaCapo Lifelong, 2004). This book came out in 1985 and is still one of the most helpful books on navigating change I've ever read.

"Tibetan Buddhists call this empty space the bardo": Yongey Mingyur Rinpoche, *In Love With the World: A Monk's Journey Through the Bardos of Living and Dying* (New York: Speigel & Grau/Random House, 2019), 50. A page-turner: will he survive his quest?

Chapter 43: Now What?

Eric Carle, *The Very Hungry Caterpillar* (New York: Philomel Books, 1969).

ACKNOWLEDGMENTS

When a writer has worked on a book for years, the list of those who helped, prodded, pushed and inspired them is lengthy. I'm sure to miss someone, but I'll do my best.

First, I must acknowledge the unsung heroes of every parent's life: those who help with childcare. I couldn't have survived those tumultuous years (1973-1980) without our beloved babysitter, Debbie Brennan, kind neighbors and friends (including Carol Lawson, the cherry pie-eating alien), and our "manny," Brad Warren. Without their assistance and moral support during the years of Edward's illness and my business launch—well, I can't even imagine where I'd be today.

My family has been my rock. My older two children, Heather and Ethan Imboden, kept me grounded through their dad's illness and my distracted floundering as a newbie entrepreneur and single parent. They put up with my eating experiments with only minor complaints. My youngest, Wylie Overstreet, has been my cheerleader, sounding board, and my most helpfully critical editor, ever pushing for more brevity and punch. My sister, Holly Tashian, read all three versions of this book, and thanks to her discerning commentary, you won't be subjected to either of the first two.

I am grateful to generous friends who read one or more drafts and gave excellent feedback: Veronika Noize, Kate McPherson, Kate Hobbie, Heather Barta, and Cassandra Sagan. Sparrow Brahe was my sensitivity reader. I've treasured the support from those who haven't given me up for lost—my dream group sisters, my virtual writing group, my color colleagues, the DIY Marketing Group, Dan Blank at WeGrowMedia and Sue Campbell at Pages & Platforms. Eternal gratitude to my best friend,

Judi Brenes, who listened to an endless litany of my writing travails and never stopped believing in me or this project.

Sometimes a stranger's actions can have far-ranging impacts. Although we've never met, KJ Dell'Antonia, formerly editor of the *New York Times* Motherlode blog, was the one who got me writing for publication again after a 20-year hiatus. Then, through the *#AmWriting* podcast she created with fellow writer Jessica Lahey, I found Sheila Athens, an Author Accelerator book coach who managed to extract 60,000 words out of me for the first draft. Nina Durfee edited the second draft (before I axed it). Another *#AmWriting* connection, my meticulous and wise editor Kim Ledgerwood at The Right Word, helped shape this final draft into something worth publishing.

Thank you to the wonderful team at Luminare Press for all of their assistance with the design, layout and publishing steps of this book, especially my very patient designer, Claire Flint Last.

From the very beginning, I envisioned a book with drawings by my friend, the prodigiously creative Kim Murton (http://kimmurton.com). Working with her was so much fun, I can't wait to do it again.

Finally, the Thin Within process would have never have become so potent without the input and wisdom of my former business partner, Judy Wardell Halliday, our gifted Thin Within seminar leaders, and the hundreds of seminar participants whose deep sharing enlightened us all.

ABOUT THE AUTHOR

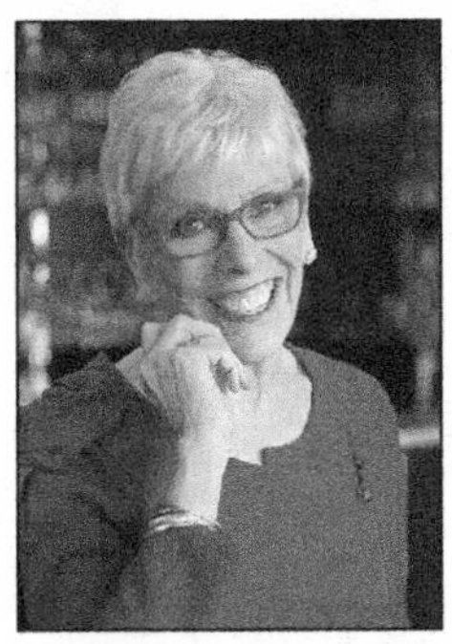

Joy Imboden Overstreet has followed her curiosity for eight decades. When she finds herself flummoxed by a problem, she figures out how to work through it, then shares the process to empower others in similar situations. This pattern is the through line in a variety of careers—guitar teacher, food writer, health educator, computer geek/tech writer, feng shui teacher and color consultant.

The Cherry Pie Paradox: The Surprising Path to Diet Freedom and Lasting Weight Loss, is based on Joy's revolutionary workshop program, Thin Within. She created it in 1975 to deal with her own weight struggles, then shared this framework for self-discovery with hundreds of others in the San Francisco Bay Area, giving participants the tools they could adapt to their own circumstances.

Joy has a Bachelor of Arts from Wellesley College, a Masters in Public Health from the University of California, Berkeley, and has yet to stop taking classes or trainings. Currently she sees clients for personal color analyses from her condo in downtown Portland Oregon. For more about that: visit www.ColorStylePDX.com.

Her articles and essays have been published in *The New York Times, Working Mother, Parents, HealthStep, Readers Digest, Computer Currents, The San Francisco Chronicle, Wellesley,* and a number of other periodicals.

During the pandemic she began a weekly newsletter, "Alive! with Joy," to cheer and encourage her readers to engage their own curiosity in seeking joy amidst life's challenges. Click the SUBSCRIBE button on her author website, joyoverstreet.com to receive it, and to hear about special events or offerings related to this book.

Made in the USA
Las Vegas, NV
18 December 2021